A TO Z OF PCOS

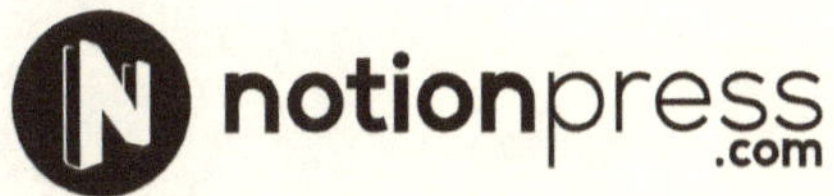

A to Z of PCOS

ALL THAT YOU EVER NEEDED TO KNOW

DR. VIMEE BINDRA | DR. SEEMA PANDEY

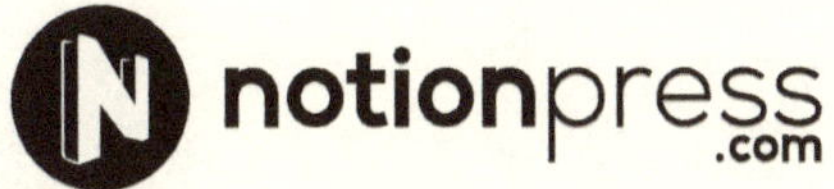

Notion Press

Old No. 38, New No. 6
McNichols Road, Chetpet
Chennai - 600 031

First Published by Notion Press 2016
Copyright © Dr. Vimee Bindra, Dr. Seema Pandey 2016
All Rights Reserved.

ISBN 978-1-946390-30-1

Illustrations by Joydeep Mitra

Dedicated to

All women worldwide suffering from PCOS, who want to stand up against it and fight back

Table of Contents

Contributors

Dr. Amita Dhakad
Consultant Gynecologist
Bombay Hospital, Indore

Dr. Amitha Indersen
Consultant Radiologist and Fetal Medicine Specialist
Apollo Cradle, Hyderabad

Dr. Asha Chandrareddy
Consultant Reproductive Endocrinology and Fertility
Bangalore

Dr. Akash Sen
DNB Gynecology
Apollo Health City, Hyderabad

Dr. Chaitanya Ganapule
Chief Endoscopic Surgeon and Consultant
Gupte and Deenanath Mangeshkar Hospital, Pune

Dr. Deepa Agarwal
Consultant Nutritionist
Apollo Cradle, Hyderabad

Dr. Kumudini Chauhan
Infertility and Laparoscopic Surgeon
Mayo Medical Centre, Lucknow

Dr. Pooja Sharma Dimri
Consultant Obstetrician and Gynecologist
Bellevue Hospital, Cloudenine Hospital, Mumbai

Dr. Prameela Sekhar
Consultant Gynecologist, Laparoscopic Surgeon
Apollo Health City
Hyderabad

Dr. Pratik Tambe
Consultant Endoscopic Surgeon and IVF Specialist
Nimriti Fertility and IVF, Thane

Dr. Rajalaxmi Walavalkar
Chief Reproductive Medicine Consultant and Endoscopic
Surgeon
Cocoon Fertility, Thane,
Mumbai

Dr. Ravi Shankar
Consultant Endocrinologist
Apollo Hospitals, Hyderabad

Dr. R N Mehrotra
Consultant Endocrinologist
Apollo Hospitals, Hyderabad

Dr. R Santosh
Consultant Endocrinologist
Magnacode, Hyderabad

Dr. Ruby K Ruprai
Consultant Laparoscopic Surgeon, Cosmetic Gynecologist
Infertility Specialist
Nice Care Medical Center, Dubai

Dr. Seema Pandey
Consultant Reprodcutive Medicine and ART Specialist
Eva Fertility Clinic and IVF Centre, Azamgarh

Dr. Tanya Buckshee Rohatgi
Consultant Reproductive Medicine and ART Specialist
Max Hospitals and NOVA IVI, New Delhi

Dr. Vimee Bindra
Consultant Laparoscopic Surgeon and
Infertility Specialist
Apollo Hospitals, Hyderabad

Foreword

Among the many health issues that women grapple with nowadays, polycystic ovarian syndrome (PCOS) is a major concern. A fairly common endocrine system disorder among women of the reproductive age, it has been estimated that around 10 million worldwide are affected by it. In India, the incidence of PCOS is 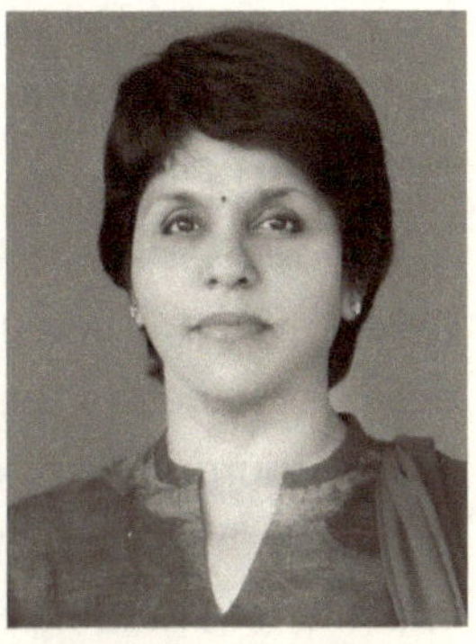 on the rise; with research indicating that nearly 35 percent of women suffer from it, a rather alarmingly high number. Yet, there is an acute lack of awareness about this condition in our society, and it often goes undetected for years.

Although a great amount of research exists in academia, very little has percolated down to the lay population in the form of books or manuals. Hence, it is commendable that Dr. Bindra and Dr. Pandey have brought together the best of available research on polycystic ovarian syndrome as a book which is interesting and easy to comprehend.

The book begins by educating its readers on the risks associated with PCOS and then it elucidates the symptoms so that self-help becomes a part of this teaching project. It also dwells on the changes that are attendant on a changing one's lifestyle, one which has been conducive to the development of this syndrome. With an attention-grabbing title, *A to Z of PCOS*, the content in the book is structured alphabetically in

26 chapters, each addressing a key aspect of the syndrome. So interestingly, chapter A is about adolescence and the challenges for a young girl to discover PCOS. Then, chapter B is about being diagnosed with PCOS and all that it entails. Progressing in this manner, every chapter continues to highlight aspects of a syndrome, one that affects one in ten women in India.

As a disorder, PCOS has social consequences, and I believe that this unique book will assist in bringing about a positive change in the way that this syndrome is regarded in the country. Also, the narrative encourages women to approach the disorder with a positive outlook and this is very important in battling PCOS and this will help the book find wide circulation and critical acclaim.

Sangita Reddy

Joint Managing Director, Apollo Hospitals

Foreword

"Whenever you read a good book, somewhere in the world a door opens to allow in more light."

Vera Nazarian

It is with great pleasure that I am writing this foreword for my dear friends' book, as they have chosen a very relevant subject and targeted it perfectly for the appropriate readers. PCOS is one of the commonest endocrine problems we see today and 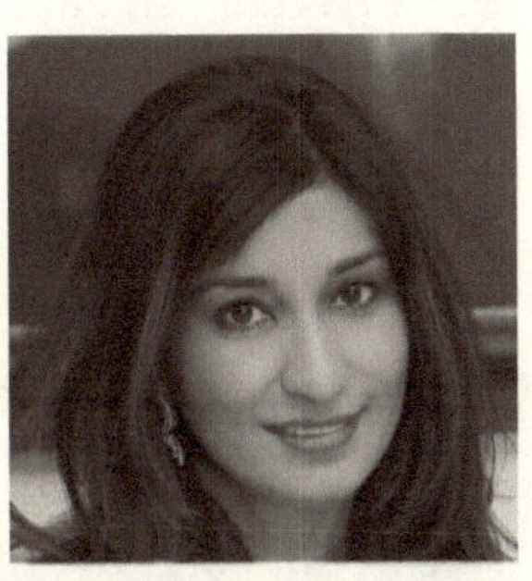 affects more than 15% of our reproductive age population. It's an enigmatic condition with multiple factors involved in its origin but the exact cause and cure is not yet known. In this era of internet, people keep searching for their symptoms online and more often than not come up with inadequate information. We need these kind of patient information books which are written by fertility specialists with a fair description of the signs and symptoms along with evidence-based management protocols so that women are not misguided.

What I really liked about this book is that it's written in a clear language and there is a touch of humor while narrating the incidents. Dr. Bindra and Dr. Pandey have taken care of every possible detail, which makes them connect with their readers directly. While reading the book, one feels as if it's their own story probably because all these stories are taken from real life day-to-day experiences.

Being a fertility specialist, a woman and the president of the federation of obstetric and gynaecological societies of India – FOGSI, I know the dire need of these kind of patient information books. In the clinic, sometimes, we are not able to answer all the queries of the patient and her relatives, so we can recommend to them to read this book if they want a wider perspective of their disease.

The concept of dividing the whole book in an alphabetical manner is really a well thought up plan. Chapters look interesting and illustrations bring a smile on your face. These illustrations are designed in such a way that they deliver the desired message while being cute and humorous.

Last but not the least, I would like to wish them success and I would recommend everyone who is directly or indirectly involved in PCOS care to read this book.

Rishma Pai

Dr. Rishma Dhillon Pai
President – Federation of Obstetric and Gyneacological societies of India
Vice President – Indian Society of Assisted Reproduction
Secretary – Indian Association of Gynaec Endoscopy

Characters

This is Meena, she is a young girl aged about twenty five years, has a lively personality with good intelligence and beautiful features. But she feels that she is obese, has excessive hair growth and acne on her face.

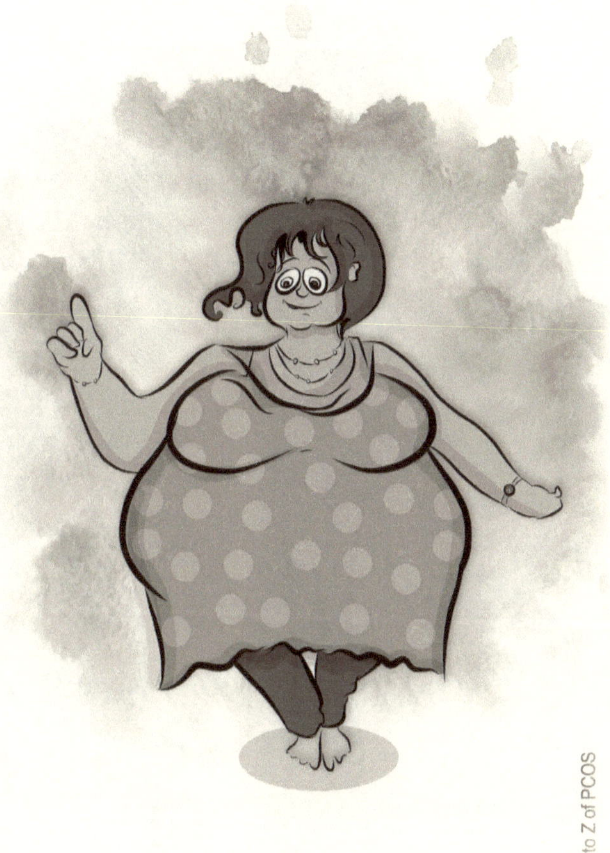

This is Maria who is very active and socially interactive, but she is confused why she has PCOS features of irregular cycles although she is not overweight.

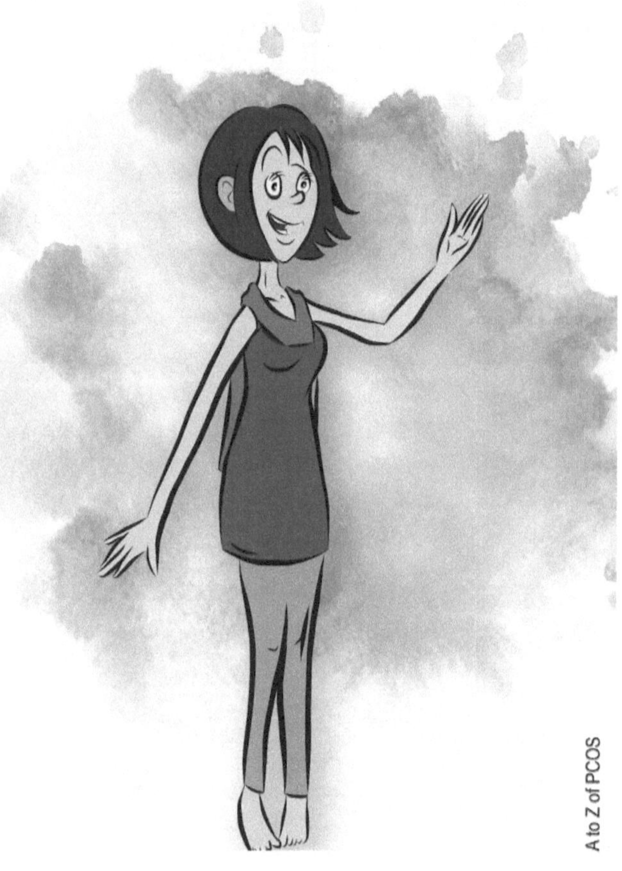

This is Mahek who studies in grade seven, she is an only child, and she loves drawing and swimming. She started menstruating a year ago. After a year of starting menstruation, she had irregular periods and started gaining weight with new appearance of acne. She is confused as to why this is happening. Is this puberty or PCOS?

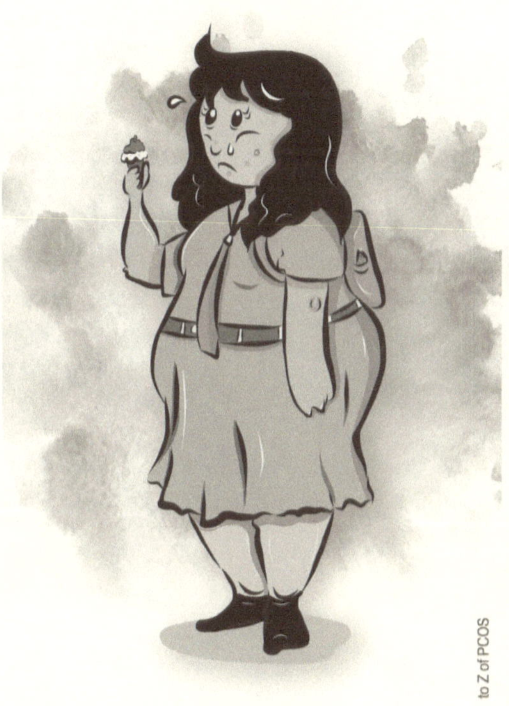

to Z of PCOS

This is Gunjan who is confused whether she is female or male as she has a long beard and hair all over.

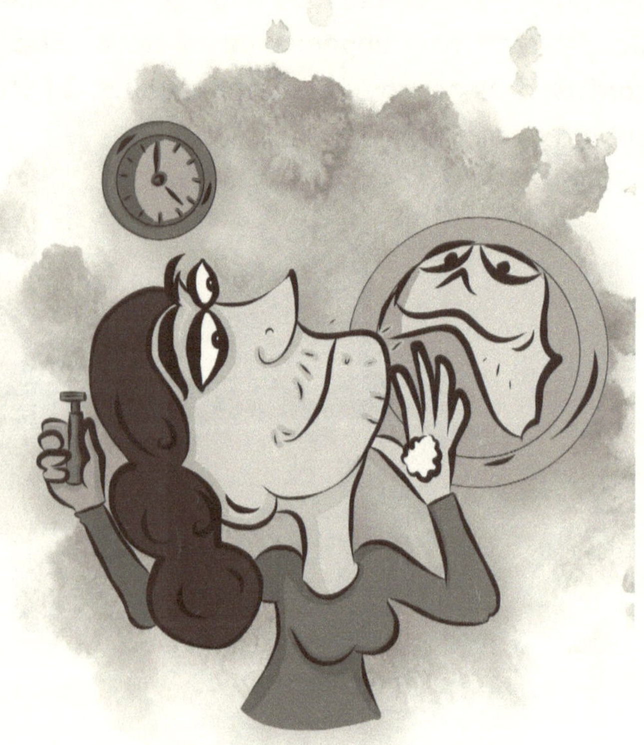

This is Deepthi, she has been married for six years and is trying to get pregnant. She is suffering from primary infertility.

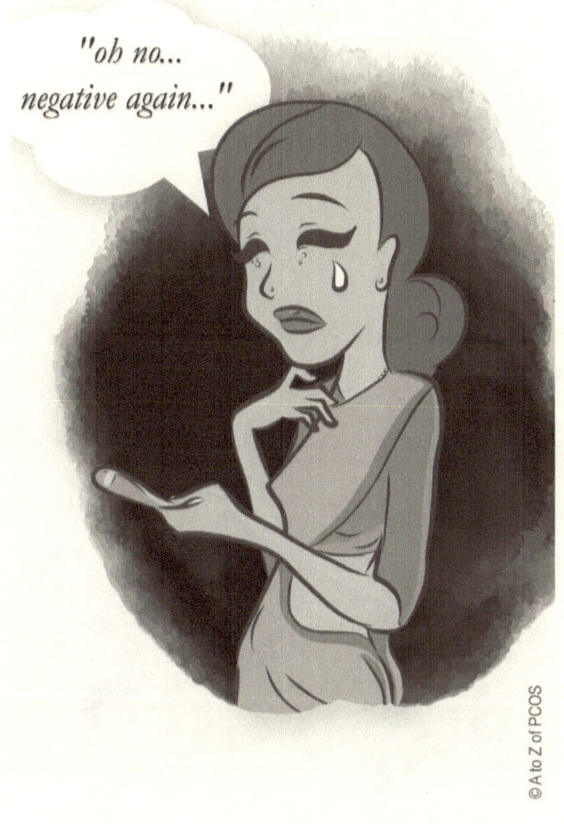

This is Harry and Peter, the most active and motile sperms who are in search of an egg for the last five years.

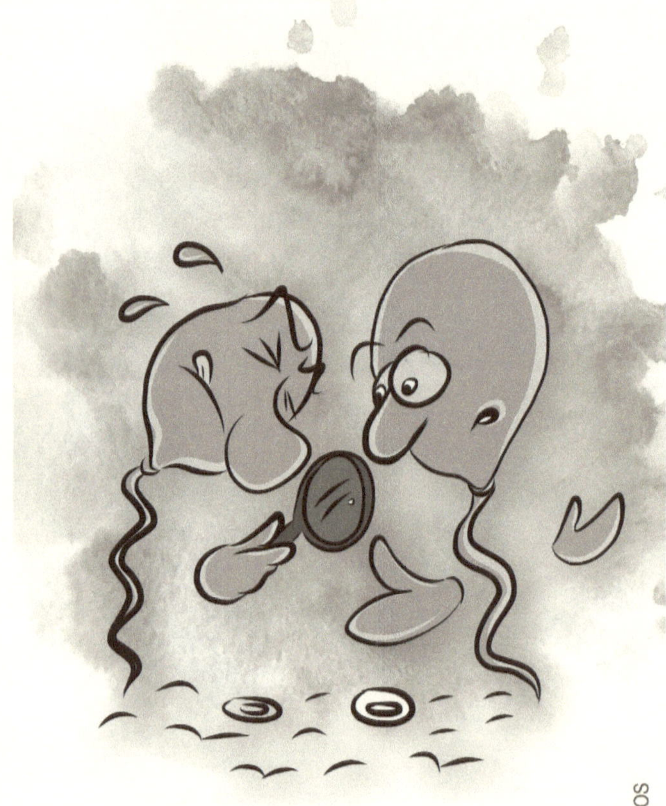

Chapter 1

Adolescence and PCOS

Dr. Tanya Buckshee Rohatgi

"Self-esteem comes from being able to define the world in your own terms and refusing to abide by the judgments of others"

Oprah Winfrey

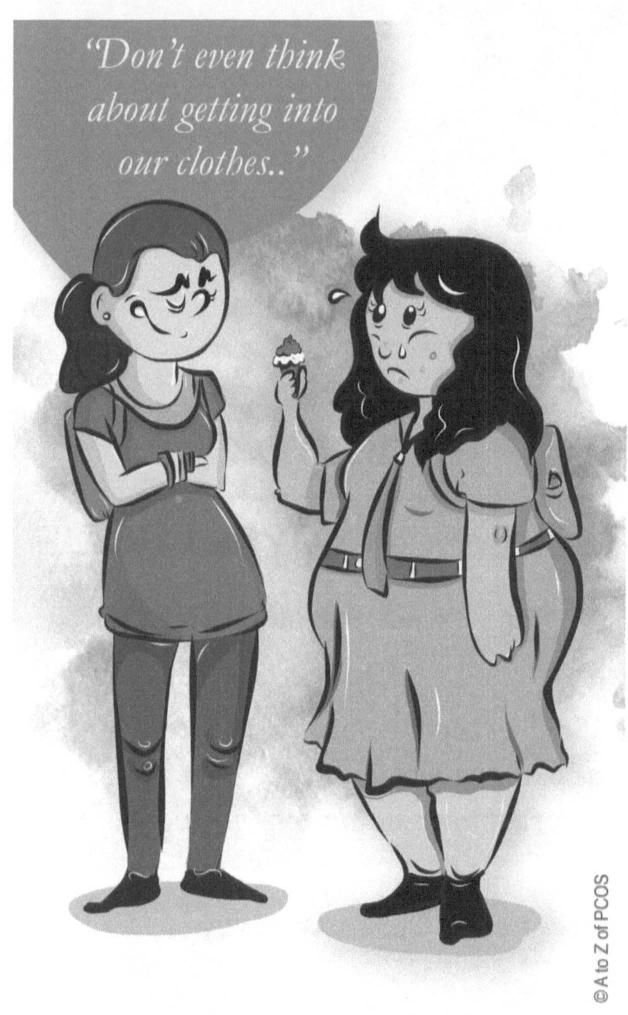

Mahek is an adolescent school going girl. After menarche she started putting on weight and had acne on her face. She was being bullied by her classmates for her appearance. Here comes the role of counseling younger girls as to how they can deal with this.

Mrs Gupta came to my clinic with Mahek her sixteen year old daughter for a check-up for her irregular periods. Mahek appeared to be a timid girl who barely made any eye contact while her mother did all the talking for her.

On closer examination, it appeared that Mahek was overweight at eighty kg with acne on her face along with excessive hair growth on her face, arms and chest.

Once we got comfortable with each other, Mahek opened up as a bright talented young girl who always came first in her class, however lately, she was being bullied at school due to her looks and all this was now affecting her studies and self-confidence.

As our consultation progressed, she suddenly blurted out, "Doctor do I have PCOS?" I was quite surprised at her knowledge of medical terms and asked her to explain the condition to me, to which she replied, she had read on the internet that it was a condition caused by an imbalance in the hormones (chemical messengers) in the brain and the ovaries.

I further explained that this was a common but an extremely variable condition in which there was excessive secretion of a hormone called luteinizing hormone (LH) (from the pituitary gland in the brain) which then causes the ovaries to make extra amounts of male hormones (testosterone) which in turn leads to irregular periods, acne and excessive hair growth in various parts of the body. The incidence in India has been noted to range between 9–36%.

Furthermore, I explained to them that early identification and treatment of PCOS will help prevent long-term consequences, which include diabetes, up to 10–fold versus the normal population, for development of type 2diabetes, high cholesterol and even cancer of the womb (uterus).

The exact cause of PCOS is unknown, however it is known to run in families, to which Mrs Gupta added that her sister was also diagnosed with PCOS.

Diagnostic Criteria

It is postulated that the syndrome begins early in childhood and may even have its onset in fetal life; however, there are no specific criteria in this age group.

Hence, to diagnose this condition in adolescence is often tricky as there is considerable overlap with physiological changes of puberty such as:

- In healthy adolescents, around 75–85% of menstrual cycles are irregular during the first year after the onset of periods (menarche). Furthermore, only approximately 40% of adolescent girls with menstrual irregularity have polycystic ovaries on ultrasound.

- Adolescents generally have increased hair growth and acne and this is a normal characteristic of puberty.

- On ultrasound examination, multiple follicular development of ovaries is a normal variant seen in adolescents.

- Transvaginal ultrasound is not feasible in a non-sexually active adolescent; and therefore, abdominal ultrasounds are recommended, and this may not be accurate especially in overweight girls. Therefore, abdominal-pelvic ultrasounds are performed in adolescents to exclude other diagnoses, and not necessarily to confirm PCOS.

Now both Mahek and her mother were surprised as they had thought that all girls with irregular periods and acne had PCOS!

So the next question Mahek raised was, "So when do we consider the possibility of PCOS and what tests and treatments are available?"

The diagnosis should be considered with a high index of suspicion in any adolescent female presenting with:

- Features as a result of high male hormones e.g. progressively increasing hair growth in male hormone (Androgen) dependent areas e.g. upper lip/chin/ upper abdomen (Hirsutism) or refractory acne.

- Menstrual irregularity which continues for > 2 years after onset of periods (Menarche).

- Personal history of early appearance of pubic hair before 8 years (Premature Pubarche), which is now known to be a precursor of PCOS.

- Strong family history of Metabolic Syndrome (high BP/ High cholesterol/ increased weight $\geq 90^{th}$ percentile for age) and/or Obesity.

In 2010 Carmina et al gave a medical diagnostic criteria for Adolescent PCOS:

1. Clinical features of hyperandrogenism or on blood tests –increased male hormones (Biochemical Hyperandrogenism)

2. Irregular periods (Fewer than eight periods per year, i.e. missing more than four periods per year / average cycle length > 45 days or < 21 days)

3. Polycystic Ovaries on Ultrasound (abdominal ultrasound ovarian volume > 10ml)

3 of the 3 above criteria

Clinical Features

Hirsutism is a key component of PCOS and is defined as excessive terminal hair growth in male hormone (Androgen) dependent areas. It should be distinguished from Hypertrichosis, which is generalized hair growth in a non-sexual distribution.

About two-thirds of adolescents with PCOS have clinical evidence of hirsutism or hirsutism equivalents which indicate high male hormones e.g. severe acne/ male pattern balding in the front of the head (Temporal Balding).

Irregular periods are also seen in about two-thirds of adolescents with PCOS, however, in adolescents this may be a normal component of puberty.

Obesity and Insulin resistance whereby body is unable to effectively use sugar due to abnormalities in the Insulin hormone that is produced by an organ in the body called Pancreas. Insulin resistance is frequently evident even in obese adolescents. In general, these adolescents have significant abdominal fat known as an "Android Distribution," even if they are not obese.

Being an inquisitive girl, Mahek asked me if these types of symptoms can be caused by some other disorders? I had to explain to her a few conditions which mimic PCOS.

Other conditions which share common features and need to be considered in the differential diagnosis include:

- Thyroid hormone abnormalities which can lead to irregular periods

- Non-classic form of congenital adrenal hyperplasia (CAH) may also present with androgen excess, irregular periods and premature pubarche. Non-classic CAH is the second most common cause of androgen excess in this age group.

- Increased Prolactin hormone abnormalities, Hyperprolactinemia results in hirsutism, irregular periods, and possibly milky discharge from the breasts (Galactorrhea). Laboratory and imaging evaluation.

So now Mahek was feeling more in control of herself and started bombarding me with questions.

Can I Do Anything to Control It?

The treatment of PCOS is as variable as its presentation and characteristics. Some components of therapy are standard while others need to be amended to fit the patient's symptoms.

Weight loss/ Lifestyle Modification

The most important treatment for PCOS is lifestyle modification; working towards a healthy lifestyle that includes healthy eating and daily exercise for about 30–60min of moderate intensity physical activity daily is recommended. Weight reduction (even 5–10% loss can lead to spontaneous resumption of menses) is indicated as first-line therapy in obese patients with PCOS.

Medical treatment is symptom based and is given to manage the particular symptoms a girl is facing like irregular periods, acne or excessive hairs.

Conclusion

In the end, I concluded by explaining to Mrs Gupta and Mahek that although recognizing PCOS in adolescents is inherently puzzling, but supporting these young girls with their lifestyle changes and medical treatments helps them not only to regain their confidence but can also assist in preventing serious long-term consequences of this disorder.

Finally a beaming Mahek left my chamber fully in charge of herself.

Chapter 2

Being Diagnosed with PCOS

Dr. Ruby K Ruprai

"No one can make you feel inferior without your consent"
Eleanor Roosevelt

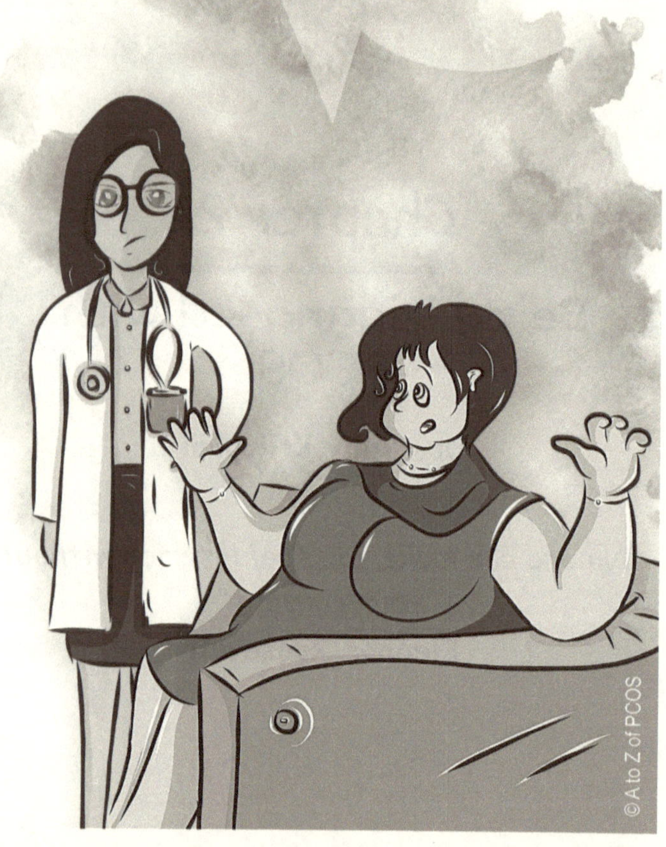

Meena went to her gynecologist and was told she has PCOS which was the reason for her gaining weight, having irregular cycles and acne. It came as a surprise to her. What was her reaction to this and how did she deal with this?

Meena visited her gynecologist two days back for her irregular periods and it came as a surprise to her that she was diagnosed with PCOS. Meena found herself wondering what this condition was and she was surprised as to how at the age of twenty five she was diagnosed with PCOS.

Meena had excessive hair growth, cystic acne, and she was heavily obese, the doctor did a few blood tests which showed high levels of testosterone and her ultrasound showed cysts in her ovaries. For the last few months, she was missing her periods frequently, had mood swings and rapid weight gain despite a rigorous exercise routine. Meena got extremely depressed. She kept building this layer of extra weight around her midsection. It was frustrating for her and difficult to deal with male pattern baldness, acne, obesity, and skin tags and now her doctor told her she had PCOS. Now how was she to deal with this?

What Is PCOS?

Many women suspect that something may be wrong when their cycle is irregular or they struggle to fall pregnant. Being diagnosed with PCOS is not easy and may come as a surprise to you. The first thing you need to know is that **you are NOT alone**. PCOS is a hormone disorder that's estimated to affect between one in 10 and one in 20 women of childbearing age, and it is the most common endocrine disorder that affects women; among young women the number is even higher, qualifying this as an epidemic.

PCOS refers to multiple cysts or fluid filled spaces in the ovaries and a host of other problems that go along with them, including anovulation (lack of ovulation) and menstrual abnormalities, hirsutism (facial hair), male pattern baldness, acne, and often obesity. Such women may also have varying degrees of insulin resistance and an increased incidence of Type II diabetes, unfavorable lipid patterns (usually high triglycerides), and a low bone density. Laboratory tests often show higher than normal circulating androgens, especially testosterone.

When the syndrome was first described in 1935 by American gynecologists Irving Stein, and Michael Leventhal, it was considered a rare disorder. Classically, PCOS was primarily considered as an infertility disorder or a cosmetic annoyance, but we now know that it is also a metabolic disorder and a serious long-term health concern. Women with PCOS are twice as likely to be hospitalized for heart disease, diabetes, mental health conditions, reproductive disorders, and cancer of the uterine lining.

Some may not show signs of the disorder until later in life, and many don't receive a diagnosis until they are struggling to get pregnant.

PCOS is a developmental disorder with genetic predilection and presents itself differently in each woman of childbearing age. PCOS has a "textbook" definition, but don't spend a lot of time over-analyzing why you're different from the next woman who has it. Every woman is different. There just isn't an answer as to why all women with PCOS are so different. For some women, symptoms emerge shortly after they begin menstruating. Others may not show signs of the disorder until later in life, or after substantial weight gain, and many don't receive a diagnosis until they are struggling to get pregnant. If a woman has fewer than eight menstrual periods a year, she probably has a 50–80% chance of having PCOS. But if she has infrequent menstruation and she has elevated levels of androgens (testosterone) in the blood, then she has a greater than 90% chance of having PCOS.

Contrary to the implication of "polycystic," some women don't have any cysts per se. A diagnosis requires only two of the following three criteria to be met; elevated levels of male sex hormones (that causes excess hair growth, acne, and baldness), irregular or absent periods, and/or at least 12 follicular cysts on one or both ovaries.

PCOS occurs when a woman doesn't ovulate, which causes a disruption in the normal cyclical interrelationship among hormones, brain and ovaries (the HPO-axis; hypothalamus-pituitary-ovarian axis).

A regular menstrual cycle.

The menstrual cycle starts when the brain sends LH and FSH to ovaries. A big LH surge is the signal that causes ovaries to ovulate, or release an egg. The egg travels down the fallopian tube and into the uterus. If the egg isn't fertilized, the lining of the uterus is shed. This is a menstrual period. After the menstrual period, the cycle begins all over again.

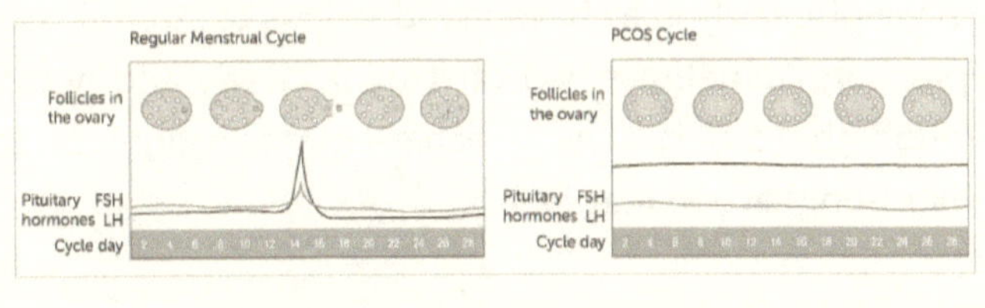

> Regular menstrual cycle vs. PCOS menstrual cycle
>
> The diagram on the left shows a regular menstrual cycle, and the diagram on the right shows a PCOS cycle with no ovulation.
>
> **What happens during a menstrual cycle with PCOS?**
>
> With PCOS, LH levels are often high when the menstrual cycle starts. The levels of LH are also higher than FSH levels because LH levels are already high, there is no LH surge. Without LH surge, ovulation does not occur, and periods are irregular.
>
> Girls with PCOS may ovulate occasionally or not at all, periods may be too close together, or more commonly too far apart. Some girls may not get a period at all.

When Missed Periods Are a Metabolic Problem

It's more than just your ovaries

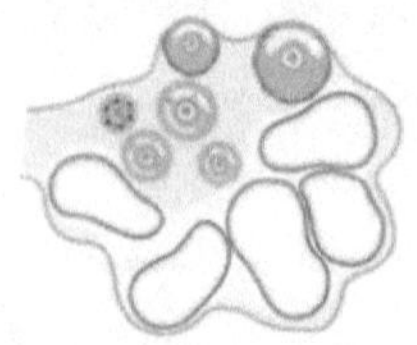

Yes, PCOS does impact ovaries. But it is also so much more than that. It is a metabolic disorder with underlying ovarian defect that impacts on just about every area of your body. You gain weight easily, may have mood swings or struggle with depression. Sometimes you can't think clearly and getting through the day is a huge achievement in light of the exhaustion that you may feel.

You may be overweight but it's not for lack of trying

Some people may look and think you are lazy, that you really should stop eating so much or that you don't care about the way you look and that's simply not true. You are often careful about what you eat. PCOS makes it so easy to gain weight and losing it is a constant struggle.

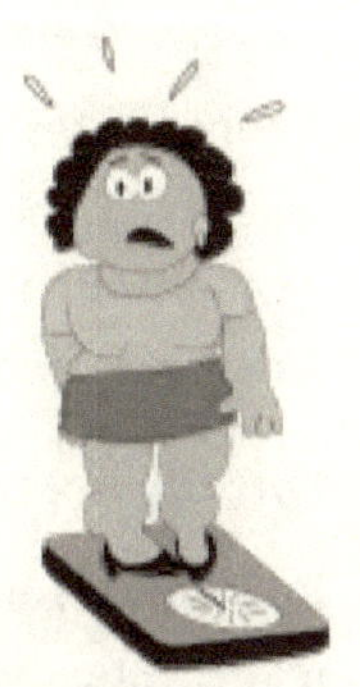

The cause of PCOS is unknown but it is thought that there is a large genetic component and if you start thinking your mother or sister may have similar symptoms that may be the case. The key features and symptoms of PCOS include anovulation and irregular menstrual cycles leading to ovulation related infertility, polycystic ovaries and increased levels of male hormones. This increase in male hormones leads to acne, weight issues, hirsutism (hair growth) and insulin resistance.

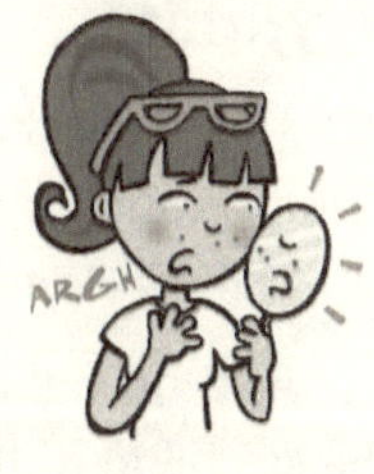

When hormone levels become disordered, the hormone insulin rises beyond healthy levels. This stimulates the production of male sex hormones, which occur naturally in all women but rise too high in women with PCOS. This can interfere with other hormones in the body that regulate everything from ovulation and conception, to hunger and weight gain. These irregular hormone levels manifest themselves in symptoms that range from irregular periods to acne to excess hair on the face, chest, and back, insulin resistance and little cysts on the ovaries (hence, the name), although you don't have to have all the symptoms to be diagnosed with the condition.

Not sure which event happens first: Higher fat stores in an obese person leading to elevated levels of insulin and insulin resistance, so perhaps weight gain leads to PCOS. On the other hand, wacky hormone levels could be messing with hunger cues, which lead women to eat more and gain weight. However, there is a small segment of women with PCOS who are of normal weight.

Insulin resistance was found in 95% of overweight women with PCOS and 75% of lean women with PCOS. Perhaps, women with PCOS have a more than 50% risk of getting Type 2 diabetes or prediabetes before age 40.

Fertility is a tricky issue

Infertility is common because it interrupts ovulation or makes it so erratic that couples can't accurately time intercourse to a woman's most fertile week.

Is Conception Impossible or Just More Difficult?

It's not impossible but it can take so much longer than the average woman. PCOS is the most common cause of infertility in women.

And now there's another thing to consider. If you do have children, it doesn't mean that PCOS doesn't affect you anymore. Remember that it affects more than just your ovaries. Because of its association with elevated insulin levels, PCOS is associated with increased risk of obesity, diabetes and cardiovascular disease.

What you can do now: In addition to modest weight loss, there are a number of pharmaceutical ways to address PCOS complications. Birth control pills can regulate menstrual cycles, diabetes drugs like Metformin can improve insulin resistance, and various fertility drugs can help women ovulate and conceive if they're struggling to get pregnant. But while these medicines can moderate symptoms or help women achieve pregnancy, none of them truly "cure" PCOS. Once you have it, you're mainly focusing on making sure you manage symptoms so it doesn't get worse. Working with your doctor to get the right combination of medicines, as well as establishing the routine of a healthy lifestyle, can prevent PCOS symptoms from worsening.

Other health issues

Because of its association with elevated insulin levels, PCOS is associated with increased risk of obesity, diabetes and cardiovascular disease. The condition tends to run in families and has been called a "cousin" of diabetes, but not all with prediabetes or diabetes have PCOS; instead, more than 50% will be diagnosed with either diabetes or prediabetes before the age of 40.

Regular menstruation is important for the prevention of endometrial cancer. Women with PCOS are three times more likely to have endometrial cancer than women without. When a woman isn't menstruating on a frequent basis, the lining of the uterus (endometrium) can begin to grow excessively and undergo atypical cell changes resulting in a precancerous condition called endometrial hyperplasia. If left untreated, this can develop into full endometrial cancer. Hormonal birth control pills are often prescribed to help women with PCOS shed their endometrium more regularly, an important measure for preventing the overgrowth of cells in the uterus.

Sometimes you just can't help it

PCOS affects more than just ovaries; moods can get altered and mood swings are not fun.

It's not convenient

There are so many women with PCOS who haven't had a natural period for months, if not years. When they do finally actually have a period, it is cause for major celebration. Not having a period for a couple of years is not convenient. It's a sign that there is something wrong.

PCOS is an expensive business

Having PCOS is an expensive business. Not only are there doctor's bills and medications, there is also the cost of fertility treatment to consider. Eating properly to manage PCOS is also crucial and healthy whole foods tend to be much more expensive than standard processed foods. So, treating PCOS is an investment of time, money and energy. It's an investment that you should be prepared to make.

PCOS is not curable

There is no cure for PCOS. One needs to make sure that they keep symptoms under control.

You are one of many

Unfortunately, PCOS affects one in ten women worldwide. Considering there are so many millions of women affected by PCOS, understanding of what PCOS is and how it affects health is important.

Get determined

PCOS is not fun and does affect every area of life. You may be at risk for a lot of secondary health issues.

Know why you need to do what you're doing

There is some very compelling evidence to explain exactly why we need to change our diets and what our new diet needs to look like.

So, Meena was just diagnosed with PCOS. Now what?

- Understand that your diagnosis is unique to you.
- Know that you're not wasting your time starting with conservative treatment of diet modification and lifestyle changes
- Remember that you are not alone.

Chapter 3

Categories in PCOS

Dr. Seema Pandey

"To accomplish great things, we must not only act, but also dream, not only plan, but also believe"
Anatole France

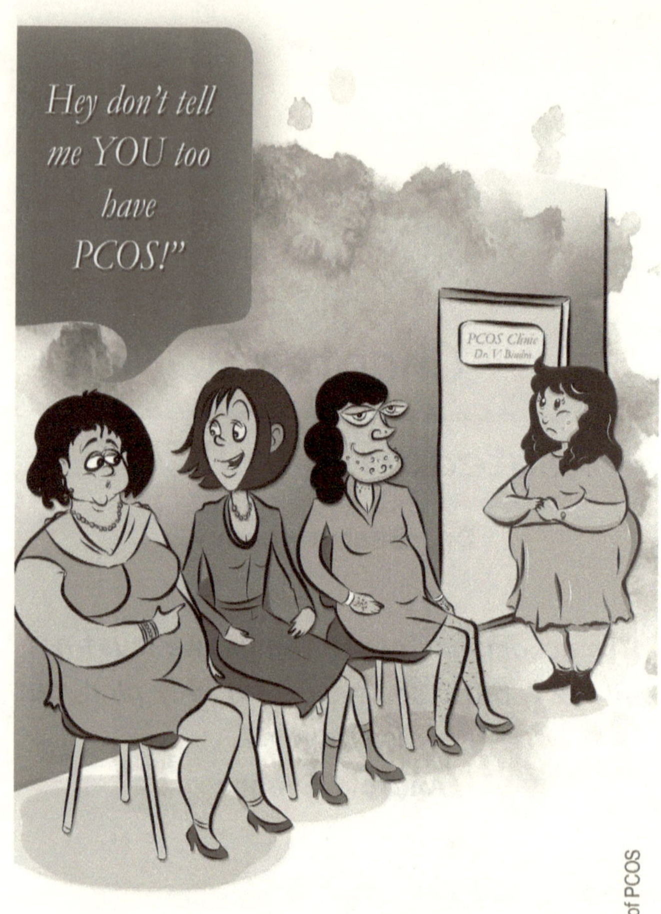

PCOS mostly is associated with obesity, but it is also seen in lean women, some have all the symptoms of PCOS other than obesity.

By reading other chapters in this book one might get confused as there is no fixed rule as to who is exactly suffering from this disease. All the explanations given by your doctor might sound confusing as a girl with 80 kg weight and body mass index (BMI)>32 might suffer from PCOS and at the same time your neighbor who hardly weighs 40 kg might also be diagnosed with the same. To make it clear I would like to talk about the criteria used for diagnosing PCOS. There are three criteria, one is oligo/anovulation (menstrual irregularity), the second is hyperandrogenism (raised male hormones in the body), and the third is polycystic morphology of the ovaries on USG (multiple cysts in the ovaries). To have PCOS you ought to have any two criteria, so if we make a permutation and combination of these three symptoms we find 4 categories or phenotypes (visual expressions) and we named them phenotype A, B, C, and D.

Phenotype A- It's also known as classic PCOS. Women having this phenotype would be having all the three components of PCOS and would be obese, hirsute and with polycystic ovaries.

Phenotype B- Also comes under classic PCOS and these women have menstrual irregularities along with raised male hormones but their ovaries look normal.

Phenotype C- This category is a milder variant as these women have regular menses and ovulate regularly but their male hormones are raised and they also depict polycystic ovaries.

Phenotype D- This is the most controversial variant of these categories and is also known as non hyper androgenic PCOS and is not included in other classifications like NIH and Andrology PCOS task force group. These women show menstrual irregularities along with polycystic ovaries but they lack the features of raised male hormones.

But looking at the various literatures and interchanging statuses of these phenotypes across the age of a single woman, this fourth group is also a part of the same disease. Though the male hormones are not raised up to the mark that they express their features physically but in a blood sample, the levels of these hormones are more than a non-PCOS woman.

What is the significance of these categories

These phenotypes vary in the degree to which they are associated with an increased risk for metabolic dysfunction and reproductive complications. The expression is also influenced by a number of determinants of epidemiology including environment (socio economic, geographic, toxicologic, lifestyle and dietary) genetic and epigenetic factors (gene variants, race, and ethnicity).

1. Metabolically phenotype A and B (classic PCOS) behave similarly, with approximately 75–85% of them demonstrating IR (insulin resistance), and some form of metabolic dysfunction. These women have an increased risk of developing glucose intolerance and diabetes mellitus. Alternatively, PCOS women with phenotype D (non hyper androgenic) who do not demonstrate overt evidence of metabolic dysfunction and are at low risk of developing disorders of glucose intolerance. Women with phenotype C (ovulatory PCOS) have levels of metabolic dysfunction and risk that are somewhat less than those with classic PCOS

but still measurably higher than those of control subjects or non hyperandrogenic PCOS.

2. Reproductively, women with ovulatory disorder will demonstrate greater degrees of subfertility than will ovulatory PCOS. Likewise PCOS women with PCOM, who are actually the vast majority of patients with the disorder, are at greater risk of ovarian hyperstimulation if treated with OI for their infertility.

Benefits of categorizing:

1. To be aware of the risks especially metabolic and cardiovascular so that one can adopt positive lifestyle changes.

2. It helps in individualizing the treatment protocol reproductively.

Chapter 4

Diabetes in PCOS

Dr. Ravi Sankar Erukulapati

"You may have to fight a battle more than once to win it."
Margaret Thatcher

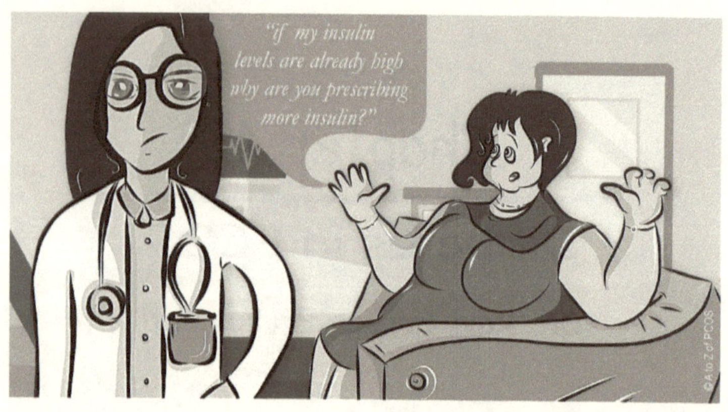

PCOS is strongly associated with diabetes and sometimes these are referred to as cousins. The cause for PCOS symptoms is mainly Insulin Resistance.

If you have been diagnosed to have PCOS and are obese, please watch your sugars, you may be suffering from deranged glucose metabolism or frank diabetes. Polycystic Ovarian Syndrome, also commonly called, PCOS is associated with many other diseases, Diabetes being one. Type 2 Diabetes, which is the common type of Diabetes is characterized by elevated blood Glucose levels and is more often seen in adult individuals who are overweight. Type 2 Diabetes is 2–4 times more common in PCOS affected women compared to women without PCOS. Around 10–20 per cent of women with PCOS will go on to develop Type 2 diabetes at some time.

Impaired Glucose Tolerance or Prediabetes, wherein blood Glucose levels are higher than normal but not as high as in those with Diabetes, is also more common in PCOS affected women. About 10–30% women with PCOS develop Impaired Glucose Tolerance at some stage in life.

Gestational Diabetes (GDM), defined as elevated blood glucose picked up first time during pregnancy is also more common in individuals with PCOS. Prediabetes, Gestational Diabetes and type 2 diabetes are more often seen in PCOS individuals if they are overweight.

PCOS and type 2 diabetes are both Obesity-related conditions that share common factors. Insulin resistance, defined as the inability of tissues in the body to use Insulin effectively, is a key factor whereby Obesity influences both PCOS and Diabetes.

About 38 to 88% of women with PCOS are overweight or obese according to one study, although PCOS can also manifest in lean women. PCOS is also associated with other features of metabolic syndrome other than Type 2 diabetes mellitus, such as elevated Blood Pressure, Dyslipidaemia and Insulin resistance. About 34 to 46% women with PCOS have Metabolic Syndrome which is a conglomeration of Obesity, type 2 diabetes, High Blood Pressure, Dyslipidaemia and Insulin Resistance.

PCOS, Insulin Resistance, Prediabetes and Diabetes

PCOS is associated with elevated levels of insulin in the blood. Insulin is a hormone that is produced by cells called Beta cells within the pancreas. Insulin regulates blood glucose levels. If glucose levels do not respond to normal levels of Insulin, body tissues become resistant to Insulin and the pancreas produces more Insulin. Excess production of Insulin is called Hyperinsulinemia and is a common phenomenon seen in PCOS as well as type 2 diabetes. Such a state when increased levels of insulin are required to maintain normal glucose levels is called Insulin Resistance and is a common feature in both PCOS and type 2 diabetes.

When blood glucose levels in the body get elevated, due to any reason including Insulin Resistance, it leads to a condition called Impaired Glucose Tolerance, otherwise called Prediabetes and if this worsens, leads to further increase in blood glucose levels and then it is called Diabetes.

Insulin Resistance and Hyperinsulinemia can occur in both normal weight and overweight women with PCOS, but more so in overweight women. Among women with PCOS, up to 35 percent of those who are obese develop Impaired Glucose Tolerance ("prediabetes") by age 40; while up to 10 percent of obese women develop type 2 diabetes as per one scientific trial. The risk of these conditions is much higher in women with PCOS compared with women without PCOS. A family history of diabetes, overweight and obesity, as well as race and ethnicity can increase the likelihood of developing Diabetes among women with PCOS.

Hence, during evaluation for PCOS, blood Glucose levels are checked along with other parameters such as Cholesterol and Triglycerides.

PCOS and Gestational Diabetes (GDM)

Some studies suggest that the risk of Gestational Diabetes (GDM) is higher among PCOS versus non-PCOS women and several studies note an increased prevalence of PCOS features in women with prior GDM. Gestational Diabetes occurs when a woman's ability to process glucose is impaired. The mother's high blood glucose levels can lead to a large baby, immature lungs, and problems for the mother and child at delivery. Among a large population of pregnant women receiving healthcare within northern California, women with diagnosed PCOS had a 2.4 fold increased odds of GDM, independent of age, race/ethnicity, and multiple gestation. GDM by itself is a risk factor for type 2 diabetes in the future.

Studies found that pregnant women with diagnosed PCOS have a more than twofold increased chance of GDM compared with women without PCOS. Further research is needed to clarify the role of obesity in mediating this association, as well as the role of infertility treatment, glucose regulating medication, and other factors during pre-pregnancy care that may impact GDM risk. Studies are also needed to determine whether PCOS women might benefit from management to reduce GDM risk and whether such measures affect pregnancy outcomes.

Once you are pregnant it is important to screen you for Gestational Diabetes during pregnancy to protect you and your baby from the deleterious effects of Gestational Diabetes. Metformin and Insulin are commonly used medications to control blood Glucose levels, along with dietary measures if Gestational Diabetes is confirmed by appropriate tests during pregnancy.

Weight Loss in Management of PCOS

Weight loss remains the main treatment for management of various problems associated with PCOS, including Glucose Intolerance and Diabetes. For example, many overweight women with PCOS who lose 5 to 10 percent of their body weight notice that their periods become more regular. Weight loss decreases Insulin resistance.

A strict diet control program and exercise regimen can help in losing the excess weight. Medications such as Orlistat can facilitate weight loss in Obese PCOS women although they have to be discontinued if planning pregnancy.

Bariatric Surgery could be considered after counseling to treat morbid Obesity in appropriate PCOS women. Weight reducing surgery can aid restoring normal menstrual cycles, reduce high Testosterone levels, improve the excess body hair, and reduce the risk of type 2 diabetes in selected women with PCOS.

If you are planning a pregnancy make sure that your sugars are well controlled, if not, then take those measures to normalize it with the help of your doctor. Lifestyle measures and an active life are the key.

Once you fall pregnant please take care of your diet and medications so that you and your baby are safe.

Chapter 5

Exercise in PCOS

Dr. Prameela Sekhar, Dr. Akash Sen

"What you do today can improve all your tomorrows"
Ralph Marston

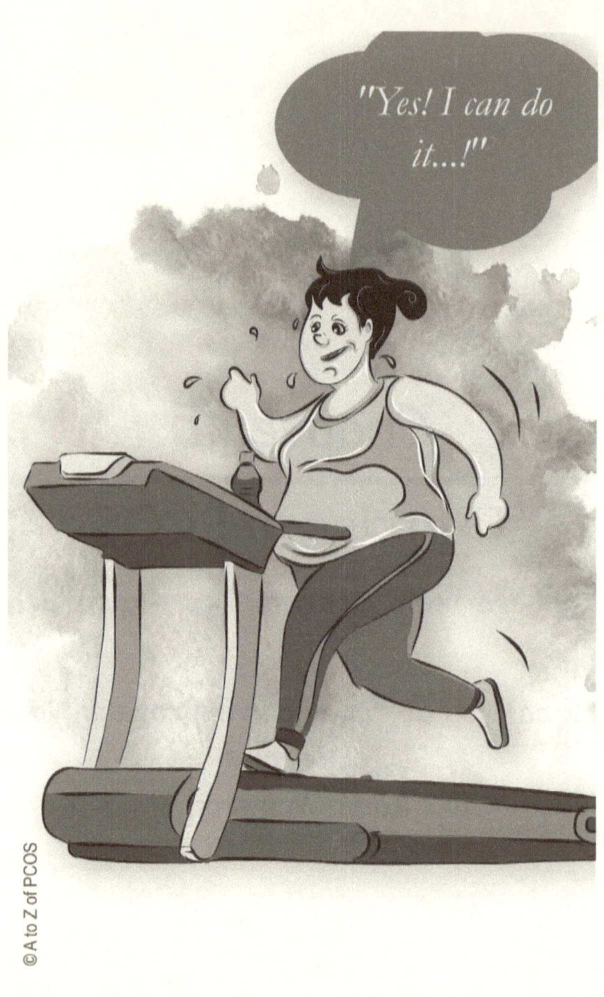

Exercise is the key to deal with your PCOS, it helps reducing insulin resistance. Even if weight loss is not happening, continue with your exercise regimen, which will help in regulating many symptoms of PCOS

"**Food** is the most abusive drug and **exercise** is the most underutilized medicine"

Whenever Meena used to visit her doctor, she used to hear from her that she needed to diet and exercise regularly and lose weight to control her PCOS symptoms. Exercise is the first line of treatment.

Exercise in PCOS Has Been Shown to Improve:

Insulin sensitivity

Frequency of ovulation

Cholesterol

Body composition

And remember, these benefits are independent of weight loss. Patient may not lose any weight while exercising but you will still feel the rewards of the above improvements. So if your doctor advices you to exercise, it's not only to lose weight but to improve your overall metabolism and hormonal imbalance.

- There hasn't been much research into the specific kinds of exercises that are beneficial for PCOS. There is a lot of information on exercise and PCOS as a whole but few suggestions of what kinds of exercises we should be doing.

- There is also a lot of research related to Type 2 diabetes and insulin resistance but these articles don't specifically look at PCOS.

- One of the main ways that exercise seems to help PCOS is the way in which it helps to manage glucose and insulin. Exercise causes glucose to be taken from the blood and moved into the muscles, lowering the need for insulin at that time and improving the body's sensitivity to insulin.

- Remember that if we can manage insulin, we will also be able to manage testosterone, the cause of a lot of PCOS symptoms.

Cardio vs. Strength Training

- *Cardio training* causes your heart rate to rise and uses energy, increasing your total calories used, which will help with weight loss. It has also been shown to lower the risk of cardiovascular disease in women with PCOS

- *Strength training*, on the other hand, builds muscle which is important in raising your basal metabolic rate so that you burn more calories while at rest and while you are exercising.

- Ideally, we should be doing a **combination** of strength and cardio training as both of these types of exercises give us different benefits.

How Much Exercise Do We Need?

- An Australian organization dedicated to providing evidence based guidelines for the management of PCOS, Jean Hailes, suggest that we should be doing **150 minutes** of exercise per week, with 90 minutes of that being moderate to high intensity aerobic exercise. So, we're looking at 30 minutes five times per week, with two of those sessions being resistance or strength training

How to Start and Sustain an Exercise Program

Finding a form of exercise that you enjoy is really important in making it sustainable. Here are some fun exercises you could consider:

- Zumba

- Pilates

- Yoga

- Aerobic classes

- Cycling

- Hiking or walking

- Swimming

WEIGHT LOSS EXERCISES

- Zumba

- Aerobic classes

- Cycling

- Hiking or walking

- Swimming

AT INITIAL STAGE OF MANAGEMENT

Yoga

- Yoga relieves stress.

- Yoga promotes weight loss.

- Yoga increases fertility.

- Yoga improves gastrointestinal balance.

Though there is no quality research available to determine the efficacy of exercise in PCOS, but in many retrospective studies on women who are on regular practice of any type of exercise for an adequate duration in each week having lesser incidence of PCOS.

Randeva et al showed that exercise, such as regular walking, reduces waist to hip ratio, an indicator of diabetes and other morbidities, and Homocystine levels, an indicator of cardiovascular risk, in overweight PCOS women.

Treatment of PCOS must focus both on normalizing short-term signs of hyperandrogenism and anovulation and on reducing metabolic complications. This can be achieved through pharmacological intervention or preferably lifestyle modification. The most preferred and effective method of treatment of PCOS is lifestyle modification. Weight loss is an important treatment strategy.

Weight loss improves practically every parameter of PCOS. In obese, anovulatory PCOS women, weight loss restores ovulation and pregnancy rates, decreases insulin levels, diminishes acanthosis nigricans, lowers testosterone levels while raising sex hormone binding globulin (SHBG) levels, and improves psychological considerations.

For obesity management, exercise is the effective way. It not only helps reduce weight but also works to improve insulin resistance and hormonal balance.

Exercise alone may not help you until you take care of your dietary habits as well.

Chapter 6

Fertility in PCOS

Dr. Seema Pandey

"Magic always happens when you direct your inner powers to the object you want to change."
Bangambiki Habyarimana

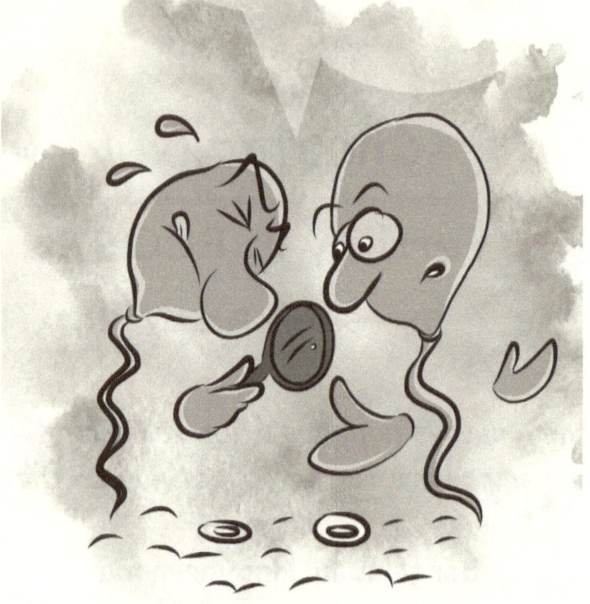

In PCOS, because of irregular cycles, ovulation is also irregular or may not happen as well. It is important to know about ovulation timing if you are trying for pregnancy.

Deepthi, a twenty one year old beautiful girl, married for two years was in my clinic with her mother, totally stressed and concerned about her ability to conceive as her periods were infrequent and scanty since she started menstruating. She was not worried about it when she was unmarried but now her husband had decided to go abroad and the family wanted her to become pregnant before he left. Looking at the mother and daughter duo, I realized that both were very pretty but almost rounded in shape and Deepthi almost looked a decade older than her age because of that extra pad of fat.

After they calmed down, I tried to talk to both of them and found that Deepthi had an elder sister whose periods were also delayed but not as erratic as the younger one and that she has also been trying to conceive for quite some time but in the middle of our conversation, her mother interrupted us telling it was not a big deal as even her periods never came on time and she has five kids. I advised them to take up a few tests before a final diagnosis and they agreed. When I scanned her, both her ovaries were full of those small cysts making it look like a spongy ball, her hormones especially thyroid (TSH) and AMH (a hormone which tells about your fertility potential and is also raised in PCOS) were dangerously high. Now it was time for a serious discussion with the family.

I told Deepthi that she was suffering from an entity called PCOS which was not exactly a disease but a group of symptoms which were the repercussions of our sedentary lifestyle. This is the common culprit in this era for causing subfertility and is on rise just like diabetes and cardiac disease. Though the exact cause as to why PCOS occurs is not known but PCOS is a familial disorder that appears to be inherited as a complex genetic trait with some genetic and epigenetic linkage as in Deepthi's family.

It's true that PCOS woman are more concerned about their fertility than their normal counterparts as for ages, regular cyclic menstruation has been associated with the potential to procure but that's not always the case. Two things which these woman have to understand is that getting your periods every month on time doesn't guarantee that you are ovulating (especially in PCOS) and at the same time getting your periods irregularly or at length doesn't make you infertile.

The raised male hormones (testosterone) and increased insulin level due to insulin resistance make these women anovulatory and menstruation infrequent. Women from different races behave differently to the same disease. It has been documented that these women when they reach their late thirties, they start menstruating more regularly than in their prime fertile years and the estimated menstrual life span of these women is extended by at least two years.

All the evidences gathered during the last seventy to eighty years have proven one thing, that PCOS women have difficulty in conceiving but once they conceive naturally, the chances of carrying the fetus till term is same as any of their friends or peers without PCOS. The result is almost the same even if you took the help of Clomid or Letrozole (Letrozole is no longer used in India).

Based on a meta-analysis done in 2006, the miscarriage rate in PCOS was similar to women with unexplained infertility but when compared to normal women it was slightly higher.

If the PCOS diagnosis is made only by the ultrasound picture of your ovaries, more than 80% chances are that no infertility treatment would be needed and spontaneous pregnancy will occur in due course of time.

Though PCOS is a leading cause of subfertility (19%) but not the sole cause, so before labeling one as sub or infertile due to PCOS, the partner's semen and other causes of infertility must be ruled out.

An interesting study done by Marita Pall and colleagues in 2004 found that there is no difference of family size between PCOS woman and normal controls although they keep suffering from chronic anovulation and suddenly a smile came to my lips as I remembered Deepthi's mother's claim regarding her kids.

Now it was time to counsel Deepthi and help her get pregnant. I told her that the first thing she needed to do was to get rid of those extra kilograms she had been carrying around, as every woman has an optimal body weight on which her cycles are regular and she ovulates, and she had to regain it. I knew it wasn't possible to do it very fast so I reassured her that even if she lost 5–10% of her present body weight more than 40% chances were that she would conceive naturally as age was on her side. Deepthi agreed to work hard and bring those changes in her lifestyle. She promised me, she would not do frequent snacking which she loves doing while watching TV. She also promised me that she would start dancing again as she used to love dancing as a small kid. I talked to her handsome husband who readily agreed to co-operate and even walk for an hour with her. They started eating less oily but tastier versions of protein and a whole grain rich diet along with green and leafy dressings as her husband loved to search for a new recipe every day for his darling wife. I prescribed her an OCpill for two cycles just to bring her hormones in range and to give enough stress-free time to lose weight and then I did not hear anything from them for a couple of months.

One fine morning, I was pleasantly surprised to find the couple in my waiting area, a thinner, prettier and much younger version of the Deepthi I knew, was beaming with a contagious smile. She told me she had missed her period that cycle and since she was feeling weird she did a home pregnancy test which turned out positive. I was overwhelmed with their joy.

Here, what I learned from her experience was that age was the strongest factor, which was on her side, younger the PCOS woman is, more are the chances that she will respond to any advised treatment, like any other normal woman so my conclusions were,

If you are diagnosed to have PCOS and are married, please plan a family at a younger age as later you may have to face more difficulties.

Weight is the worst kind of co-morbidity which makes your symptoms worse as it indirectly promotes the synthesis of male hormones in your body so try to get rid of it as fast as possible.

Lifestyle management is the key, along with right advice regarding regaining the balance of your hormones may make you pregnant naturally.

If you have tried all these methods and none are working for you please take the help of your reproductive medicine expert who knows you and your symptoms well.

Try to reduce the level of stress and don't fight it alone, try to talk to your partner, if he is not helping take the support of helping groups and keep your thoughts positive, that way you will not release those stress hormones which make your condition worse.

Last but not the least; never concentrate on being infertile or less feminine because of PCOS.

Chapter 7

Goal of Treatment in PCOS

Dr. Ruby K Ruprai

"Every goal first started as something in our mind. You have it all within you"
Deborah Day

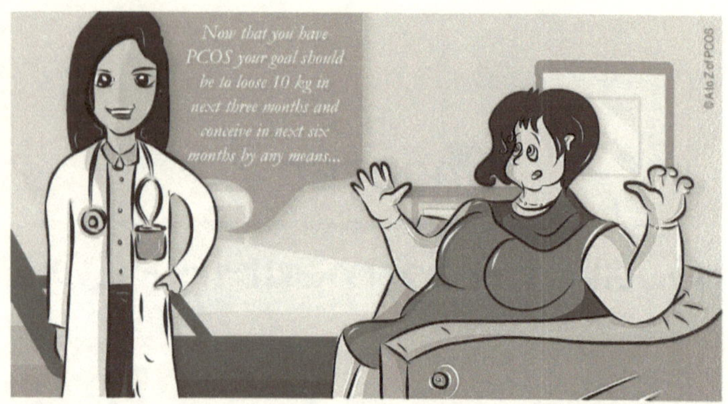

I have PCOS. What is the treatment for PCOS? What can I do to prevent complications?

PCOS cannot be cured but with your determination and hard work, you can conquer this syndrome and keep it suppressed.

WHAT CAN YOU DO ABOUT YOUR PCOS?

Let's begin!!!!

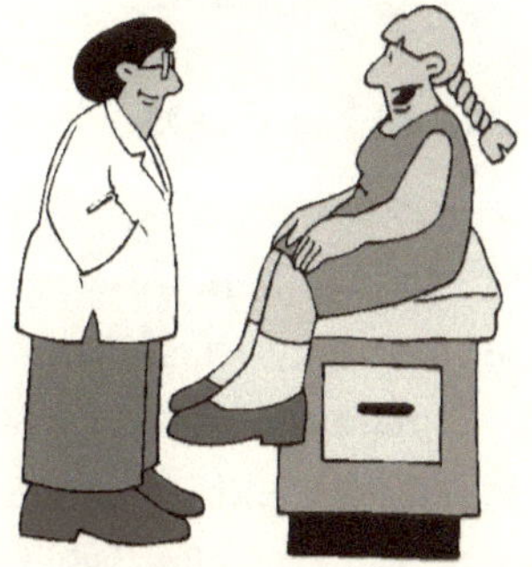

There is no cure for PCOS, but there are ways to keep it in check. Treatment goals are based on your symptoms; some women require a combination of treatments. If you have PCOS, get your symptoms under control at an earlier age to help reduce your chances of having complications like diabetes and heart disease. Talk to your doctor about treating all your symptoms, rather than focusing on just one. Also, get tested for diabetes regularly. Other steps include:

- Eating right
- Exercising
- Not smoking

Goal of treatment in a PCOS woman varies as per the stage of life when she has been diagnosed with it. For example, the treatment plan would be different for a 17 year old girl whose main concerns are her erratic periods, body image and acne. The same girl, when she becomes 20 plus and is married, her prime concern would be fertility and she would think of getting pregnant as soon as possible. We will have to revise our strategy for a woman who is in her 30s and has completed her family. Here our focus would be to save her from dreadful metabolic consequences like diabetes, hypertension and cardiac problems.

Medical Treatment for PCOS

Medical treatment for PCOS varies depending on your unique situation and the management of your main individual concerns, such as infertility, hirsutism, acne or obesity. Birth control pills regulate menstrual cycles, Metformin can improve insulin resistance, and various fertility drugs can help women ovulate and conceive. While these medicines can moderate symptoms or help women achieve pregnancy, none of them truly "cure" PCOS. Working with your doctor to get the right combination of medicines, as well as establishing the routine of a healthy lifestyle, can prevent PCOS symptoms from worsening.

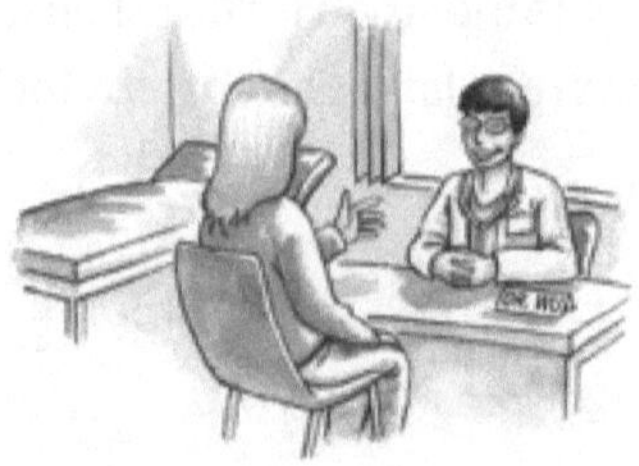

Medications

Your doctor may prescribe a medication to:

- Regulate your menstrual cycle
- Help you ovulate and get pregnant
- Reduce excessive hair growth

Regulate your menstrual cycle. If you are not trying to conceive, combined birth control pills (containing estrogen and progestin or anti-androgen) can be used to regulate your cycle. The hormones often help keep cysts at bay and cycles regulated. Whilst on the pill, your cycle will be regular and many symptoms of PCOS will be managed. These pills decrease androgen production and give the body a break from the effects of continuous estrogens, lowering your risk of endometrial cancer and correcting abnormal bleeding. Most contraceptive pills regularize periods but some (Diane) are also specifically beneficial for hirsutism. As an alternative to birth control pills, you might use a skin patch or vaginal ring that contains a combination of estrogen and progestin.

If you're not a good candidate for these pills, an alternative would be to take progesterone for 10–14 days every one to two months. This therapy regulates periods and offers protection against endometrial cancer, but it doesn't improve androgen levels and it won't prevent pregnancy. The progestin-only (Minipill) or progestin containing intrauterine device (Mirena) are better choices if you also wish to avoid pregnancy. Natural progesterone should be the basis of PCOS treatment, along with attention to stress, exercise, and nutrition. The disappearance of facial hair and acne are usually obvious signs that hormones are becoming balanced, but this can take at least six months, in conjunction with proper diet and exercise. If your symptoms return, stay on the full dose for six more months. But, progesterone alone does not help reduce acne and hair growth.

Your doctor may also prescribe metformin that improves insulin resistance and lowers insulin levels. This drug may help with ovulation and lead to regular menstrual cycles. Metformin also slows the progression to type 2 diabetes if you already have prediabetes and aids in weight loss if you also follow a diet and an exercise program. It must be taken with a healthy diet and can have some negative side effects. Keep in mind that Metformin really pairs best with a low-glycemic index lifestyle, so if you go on it, consider making a huge change in how you eat as well.

How birth control pills help

- Correct the hormone imbalance

- Lower the level of male hormones/ testosterone (which will improve acne and lessen hair growth)

- Regulate your menstrual periods

- Help clear acne

- Lower the risk of endometrial cancer (which is slightly higher in young women who don't ovulate regularly)

- Prevent an unplanned pregnancy if you are sexually active

Keep in mind as soon as you stop taking the medication, your symptoms may return. Therefore it is imperative that you maintain a healthy lifestyle as discussed above and use the medical treatment as a means to jump-start your treatment.

Help you ovulate. Lack of ovulation is the most common cause of fertility problems in women with PCOS. In overweight women with PCOS and anovulation, diet adjustment and weight loss are associated with menstrual regulation and ovulation.

- If you're trying to become pregnant, you may need a medication to help you ovulate. Other reasons for infertility in both the woman and man should be ruled out before fertility medications are used. Once other causes have been excluded, the first-line medication to stimulate ovulation is clomifene citrate.

- If clomiphene alone isn't effective, your doctor may add Metformin (Glucophage) with clomiphene. The combination may help women with PCOS ovulate on lower doses of medication. Metformin makes the body cells more sensitive to insulin and lowers testosterone production. In addition, metformin treatment has been shown to improve hirsutism, acne, and menstrual irregularities in thin PCOS women. Recent research has shown metformin to have other positive effects, such as decreased body mass and improved cholesterol levels.

- If you don't become pregnant using clomiphene and metformin, your doctor may recommend using gonadotropins — follicle-stimulating hormone (FSH) and luteinizing hormone (LH) injections. Another medication that your doctor may have you try is Letrozole. Both clomifene and gonadotrophins are associated with risk of multiple births although the risk is higher with gonadotrophins. When taking any type of medication to help you ovulate, it's important that you work with a reproductive specialist and have regular ultrasounds to monitor your progress and avoid problems.

- Treatment by IVF is another option.

Reduce excessive hair growth and/or acne. For women requiring contraception, your doctor may recommend birth control pills (oral contraceptives) that help in reducing excessive hair growth. Commonly used is the Diane (cyproterone acetate) that has anti-androgenic effects that blocks the action of male hormones that contribute to acne and growth of unwanted hair.

Other Anti-androgen medications such as, spironolactone blocks the effects of androgens on the skin and reduce abnormal hair growth in women and make hair lighter and finer. However, it can take up to 6–8 months to see an improvement. Because spironolactone can cause birth defects, effective contraception is required when using the drug and it's not recommended if you're pregnant or planning pregnancy/ breast feeding. Finasteride has the same effect. In women with insulin resistance, diabetes or obesity, metformin by reducing insulin resistance can minimize abnormal hair growth. Eflornithine is a cream which is applied to the face and acts directly on hair follicles to inhibit hair growth.

Electrolysis or laser treatments are faster and more efficient alternatives than medical therapy. Anti-androgens are often combined with birth control pills. These medications should not be taken if you are trying to become pregnant.

> - **Treatment for acne** includes the birth control pill, topical creams, oral antibiotics, and other medications.
>
> - **Treating hair growth.** Options include bleaching, waxing, depilatories, spironolactone, electrolysis, and laser.

Surgery

- Laparoscopic 'ovarian drilling' (puncture of few small follicles with electrocautery) is sometimes used and often results in spontaneous ovulation or indeed ovulation after adjuvant treatment with clomifene or FSH. It's sometimes used when a woman does not respond to fertility medicines. This procedure carries a risk of developing scar tissue on the ovary. This surgery can lower male hormone levels and help with ovulation. But, these effects may only last a few months. This treatment doesn't help with loss of scalp hair or increased hair growth on other parts of the body.

- Bariatric (weight loss) surgery may be effective in resolving PCOS in morbidly obese women. Morbid obesity means having a BMI of more than 40, or a BMI of 35–40 with an obesity-related disease.

Support

Having PCOS can be difficult. You may feel:

- Embarrassed by your appearance

- Worried about being able to get pregnant

- Depressed

Getting treatment for PCOS can help with these concerns and help boost your self-esteem. You may also want to look for support groups in your area or online to help you deal with the emotional effects of PCOS. You are not alone and there are resources available for women with PCOS. Finding good support is vital to managing your PCOS.

Remember, staying motivated is the key because there is no cure for PCOS but its symptoms can be treated, and the chance of getting diabetes or heart disease can be lowered.

You Are Not Alone

Remember that. There is an entire community online, between bloggers, You Tubers and message boards, of women suffering from PCOS and sharing their stories. Many come with pregnancy success, which is awesome, and some don't. Please reach out if you're looking for support, advice, or just someone to talk to.

Having a healthy lifestyle through ups and downs is the first step to living well with PCOS!

Stay positive! It can take time to lose weight. Remember that taking care of yourself by eating right is a success even if you don't see a big change in your weight.

Chapter 8

Hirsutism in PCOS

Dr. Vimee Bindra

"Your attitude is like a box of crayons that color your world. Constantly color your picture gray, and your picture will always be bleak. Try adding some bright colors to the picture by including humor, and your picture begins to lighten up."
Allen Klein

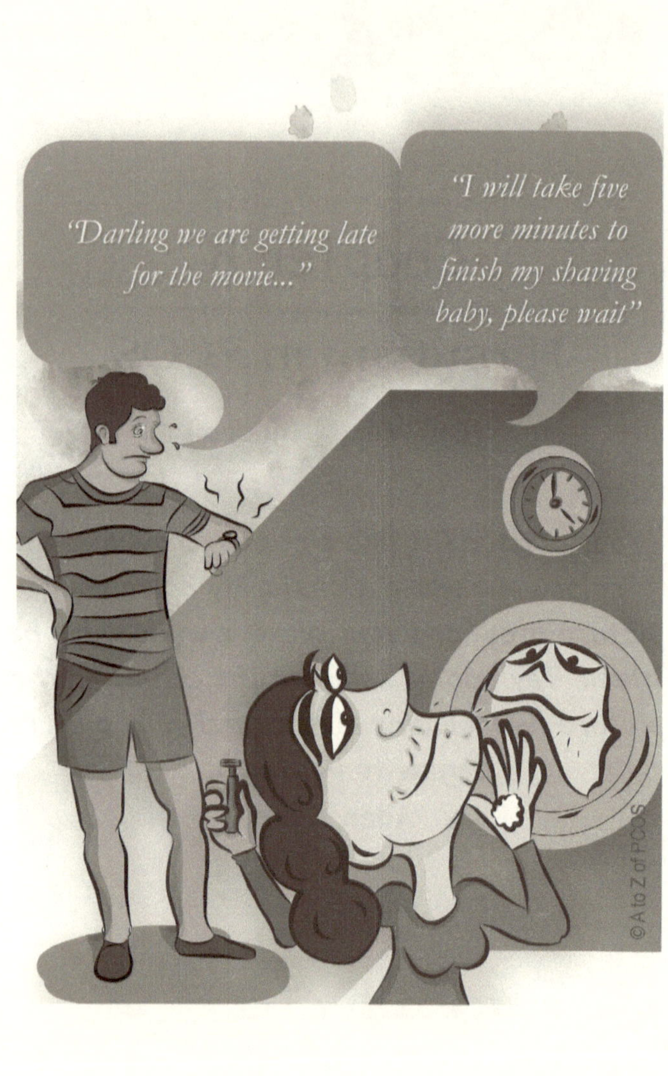

"Darling we are getting late for the movie..."
"I will take five more minutes to finish my shaving baby, please wait"
©A to Z of PCOS

She was depressed, she used to feel lonely, and she started avoiding meeting her friends as her fiancée had broken up with her. Would you like to know the reason? The reason was her appearance, as she had started getting thick coarse hair everywhere; she had a moustache and hair in the beard area and everywhere else such as thighs, back, upper chin and abdomen. Do you know what she was suffering from? She was suffering from Hirsutism which happens in PCOS due to excess of male hormones. Let's see how you can deal with this condition.

Hirsutism is the excessive hair growth of facial or body hair in women. Hirsutism can be seen as coarse, dark hair that may appear on the face, chest, abdomen, back, upper arms, or upper legs. PCOS, in which ovaries produce excess androgens, is the most common cause of hirsutism and may be seen in up to 10% of women. Hirsutism is generally slowly progressive in onset in PCOS. The Ferriman-Gallway scoring system is a useful method of quantifying hirsutism. In this system, a score (ranging from 0 for no growth to 4 for extensive growth of terminal hair) is assigned to the following body areas:

Upper lip
Chin
Chest
Upper back
Lower back
Upper abdomen
Lower abdomen
Upper arms
Thighs

This is a very depressing symptom for the patients with PCOS as it tends to change their appearance. It even leads to feeling of rejection and social withdrawal and needs to be handled carefully.

There are a variety of medical and cosmetic treatments available for hirsutism that your doctor may advice.

Medications

Birth control pills

Androgen receptor blockers Eflornithine cream

Spironolactone

Flutamide

Finasteride

GnRH analogues only for severe forms.

Cosmetic Treatments

Shaving

Plucking

Waxing

Bleaching

Depilatory agents

Laser

Electrolysis

Birth control Pills are the most commonly suggested treatment. It inhibits ovulation and increases sex hormone binding globulin and decreases androgens. It has the added advantage that it helps regulating cycles and protects against unwanted pregnancies.

Anti-androgenic Medications

Spironolactone, a *diuretic* or "water pill," often is prescribed in combination with birth control pills. It has been found to directly block the effects of androgens in hair follicles and has been used to treat hirsutism. Side effects may include dry skin, heartburn, headaches, irregular vaginal bleeding, and fatigue. More than two-thirds of the women on high dose spironolactone will have a significant decrease in hirsutism. Other anti-androgenic medications include *flutamide*, which blocks androgen receptors, and *finasteride*, which blocks the conversion of testosterone to more active androgens. Side effects can include rare but harmful effects to the liver.

Cosmetic Therapy

Cosmetic removal of hair in women with hormonally associated hirsute such as PCOS always should be accompanied by medical therapy in order to be successful.

Temporary Hair Removal

For temporary treatment of mild hirsutism, many women pluck unwanted hairs. However, plucking tears the hair from its living follicle and can irritate sensitive skin. Waxing carries the same risks of irritation and infection, especially in androgen sensitive areas. Depilatories are chemicals that dissolve the hair shafts and may cause irritation to sensitive facial skin. Bleaching can be used in small areas of the body, particularly the upper lip, to make excessive hair less noticeable, but excessive bleaching should be avoided.

Although not satisfying to many women, shaving is probably the simplest and safest way to temporarily remove hair. Because of the continued growth of the hair, shaving is required frequently and may result in irritating stubble, but an electric razor may produce less skin irritation than a blade. Shaving seldom has medical side effects.

A facial cream containing *eflornithine hydrochloride* may be used in combination with the previously mentioned cosmetic therapies to slow the growth of excessive facial hair. Some women have worsening of acne with eflornithine use. Its safety in pregnancy or effectiveness on other body parts has not been established and should not be used.

Permanent Hair Removal

There are two types of permanent hair removal: electrolysis and laser treatment. During electrolysis, a very fine needle is inserted into the hair follicle. A mild electric current is sent through the needle to permanently destroy the hair follicle's ability to produce hair. It is used only for small areas on the body.

Laser treatments may be used on large areas of the body, although their long-term effectiveness is not as well documented as electrolysis. During laser hair treatment, a beam of light is passed through the skin to the hair follicle to destroy it. People with light skin and dark hair usually achieve the best results with laser hair removal.

Both methods of hair reduction are moderately painful, depending on the area of skin being treated, and multiple treatments usually are required. Nevertheless, electrolysis and laser are very effective ways to remove unwanted hair. However, they may not reduce all hair growth and may not always be permanent. Without concurrent medical treatment, new hair will grow. It is best to delay laser or electrolysis treatment for at least 6 months after beginning medical treatment so that the growth of new terminal hairs will be reduced.

What to Expect From Treatment of Hirsutism

Hormone treatment generally prevents new terminal hairs from developing and may slow the growth rate of existing hairs. Generally about 6 months of hormone therapy is required before the rate of hair growth decreases significantly. Once a hormone treatment has proven to be effective, it may be continued indefinitely. Electrolysis or laser can remove any hair remaining after hormone therapy. Because it usually is not possible to cure the hormonal problem that causes hirsutism, ongoing medical treatment is required to manage it. Hirsutism will frequently return if medical treatment is stopped. Sometimes a combination of treatment methods is needed for best results.

Dealing with hirsutism and PCOS can be emotionally difficult. You may feel unfeminine, uncomfortable, or self-conscious about your excessive hair growth or weight, as well as worried about your ability to have children. Even though you may be embarrassed to share these feelings with other people, it is very important to talk with your physician as soon as possible to explore the medical and cosmetic treatments available to treat these disorders. It also is important for you to realize that these are very common problems experienced by many women and you are not alone.

Hirsutism is a common disorder that usually can be treated successfully with medication. Following medical treatment, electrolysis or laser treatment can be used to permanently reduce or remove any remaining unwanted hair. If other female family members have experienced excessive hair growth, you should watch for early signs of hirsutism in yourself and your children, especially during adolescence. Hirsutism is frequently a result of PCOS. Both hirsutism and PCOS are easier to treat when diagnosed at a young age.

Yes it affects your appearance but is it only external beauty that matters?

Beauty is how you feel inside, and it reflects in your eyes. It is not something physical

- Sophia Loren

Chapter 9

Insulin Resistance in PCOS

Dr. R Santosh

"Change your thoughts and you change your world"
Norman Vincent Peale

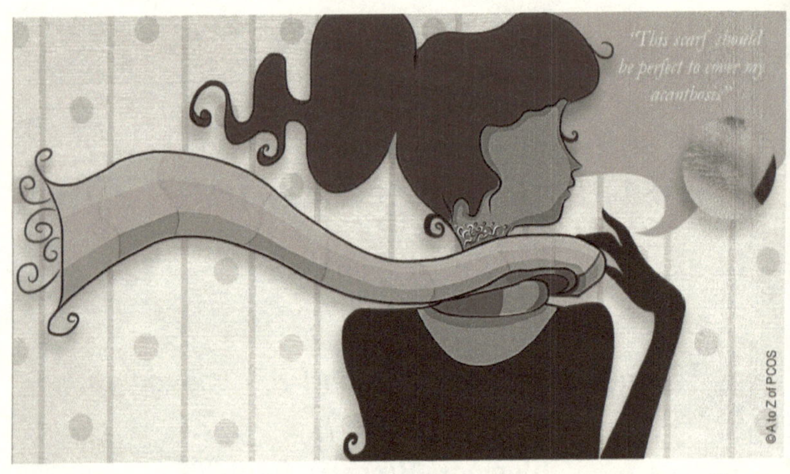

Insulin resistance affects all metabolic factors and also affects skin by causing some skin tags and darkening of skin at the neck area called as Acanthosis Nigricans.

Insulin Resistance and PCOS

Insulin resistance seems to be the key factor that contributes to Polycystic ovarian syndrome.

What is insulin?

Insulin is a hormone that pushes the glucose from the food that we eat into the cells of the body. When we eat food, it's broken down into small nutrients especially glucose, fats and amino acids. Insulin is a hormone that is released from the pancreas immediately after food is ingested. It immediately moves the glucose into the cells of the brain, muscle, heart, liver, kidneys and other essential organs.

What is insulin resistance?

Insulin resistance is the inability of insulin to push the glucose into the cells due to a problem with its receptors.

Does that mean you have diabetes?

No. Usually the body compensates by producing more insulin. Therefore the blood sugar remains normal, although to keep it normal, insulin levels are higher than those who don't have insulin resistance.

If the insulin levels have compensated for the insulin resistance, then why should I worry at all?

There are two things to worry about:

1. There are certain areas of the body that are not insulin resistant and they get harmed.

2. After a while, especially in the late thirties and early forties, the pancreas get tired of producing high levels

of insulin and finally starts to not function well. When this happens, blood glucose starts to rise and a person progresses into prediabetes and then frank diabetes.

What causes the insulin resistance in the first place?

1. The strongest risk factor is genes. Insulin resistance occurs in those people who have family members with insulin resistance; that is diabetes or PCOS. Even if the parents themselves don't have diabetes, other family members having diabetes or PCOS increase the risk of insulin resistance.

2. Lack of exercise: Lack of exercise is one of the important contributors to insulin resistance. Exercise improves the muscle blood flow and improves the action of insulin.

3. Eating carbohydrate and simple fat rich food. Eating such food not only worsens the insulin resistance, but also requires more insulin to be secreted after it, thereby tiring the pancreas early.

4. Mental stress. It causes some hormonal changes in the body, which worsen the insulin resistance.

What are the areas that are not insulin resistant? How does that matter?

The three areas that are classically not insulin resistant are:

1. **Skin:** Insulin directly acts on certain areas of the skin. It causes darkening, thickening and folding of skin near the neck (starting from behind the neck and slowly progressing to encircle it), the underarms, the elbows, the knees and the pubic areas. This is called acanthosis

nigricans which is the hallmark of a patient having insulin resistance. Severe degrees of insulin resistance also cause skin tags in these areas.

2. **Truncal fat.** Insulin directly acts on these areas to increase the fat on the trunk. Those with insulin resistance tend to put on weight over the shoulders, chest, hips, abdomen, arms and thighs. The areas below the elbow and below the knee are generally lean.

3. **Ovaries.** Insulin directly acts on the ovaries and causes cyst formation. It also increases the free male hormones in the blood. The polycystic ovaries release female hormones irregularly (irregular menses, infertility) and increased male hormones (acne, hair fall, and unwanted hair growth)

How can we reduce insulin resistance?

1. **Dietary modifications**

    a. Number of meals: Eating small and frequent meals will make sure you do not put a load of glucose at a given point of time hence your body releases little insulin. Eat six meals rather than three meals a day.

    b. Protein helps insulin work better, eat 1g/kg body weight (IBW) everyday. Include lean meats, egg whites, pulses, legumes for protein.

    c. Eat complex carbohydrates like whole grains, single polished rice and legumes over simple carbs like maida, bakery products, and fruit juices.

    d. Limit the amount of fat intake; avoid reusing of oil and usage of vanaspati, lard and margarine.

2. **Exercise**

Doing at least 150 minutes per week of aerobic exercises improves muscle blood flow and improves insulin resistance. There must be no more than one day gap between two days of exercise. We should walk as briskly as possible, but should not become breathless, and should be able to speak to the person who is exercising with us.

3. **Pranayama**

Simple breathing exercises bring down the stress hormones and improve the insulin resistance drastically.

4. **Medication**

There are simple and safe medicines like metformin and myoinositol that help reduce insulin resistance, however they have to be prescribed only by your treating doctor.

Chapter 10

Juggling with your Hormones

Dr. Chaitanya Ganapule

"Life is juggling act with your own emotions. The trick is to always keep something in your hand and something in the air."
Chloe Thurlow

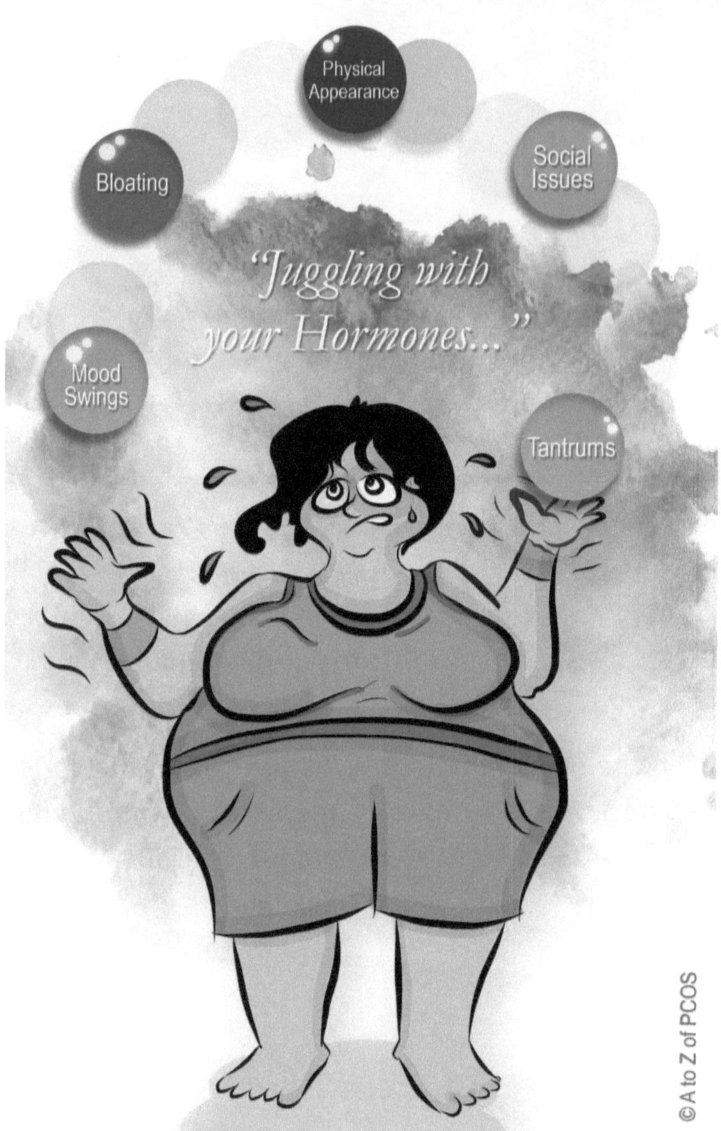

Woman is always known to be a multi-tasker. Believe me or not, they are real multi-taskers and if they have PCOS they are handling too many things at a time.

Why only women? Whether its pre-menstrual syndrome or PCOS, they show their tantrums to women only, why are men spared? I think every woman asks this question whenever they face these hormonal effects. Everybody has hormones then why it affects only women is a mystery unsolved for ages.

Women are known multi-taskers in terms of work, entrepreneurship, homecare, childcare, and also tactfully dealing with her hormones. She should be conferred some PhD or doctorate on how to handle multiple things with ease.

PCOS is associated with many consequences like irregular periods, excessive hair growth, acne, infertility and so on. It becomes imperative to know what happens exactly in our body when one suffers from PCOS.

To understand the changes that take place in our body in PCOS, we must first understand how one gets her normal periods. "Periods" are the external manifestation of a major juggling of hormones that takes place in the body. The three most important organs that play a role in normal menstruation are – Brain, Ovaries and Uterus. Two important areas of the brain play a vital role in normal periods and those are the hypothalamus and the pituitary gland.

"Hormones" are the substances that are secreted by specialized glands of the body and carry signals from one organ to the other.

The hypothalamus secretes a hormone called as gonadotropin releasing hormone (GnRH) that acts on the pituitary gland. In response, the pituitary gland secretes two hormones called as follicle-stimulating hormone (FSH) and luteinizing hormone (LH). These hormones are then carried to the ovary and bring about development of the egg. The developing egg produces two hormones called as Estrogen and progesterone (popularly known as" female hormones"). Estrogen and Progesterone then act on the uterus and bring about development of the lining of the uterus called as "Endometirum".

This entire juggling of hormones takes place with the sole objective of achieving pregnancy. If pregnancy doesn't takes place, endometrium is shed off, what we call as "periods".

In women suffering from PCOS, this juggling of hormones is altered and that produces the classical symptoms of PCOS.

But what exactly happens in PCOS? Let's try and understand the complex changes that occur in PCOS.

The frequency at which GnRH is secreted is increased in patients with PCOS. The increased frequency of PCOS causes pituitary to secrete more of LH and less of FSH. This leads to a "LH" dominant environment in the ovary.

LH dominant environment makes the egg secrete more of androgens (Male Hormones) and prevents the development of the egg. As the development of the egg is jeopardized, the chances of conception are also reduced and the lady suffers from "infertility".

Due to excess secretion of male hormones, there is excessive hair growth seen on the face and other parts of the body termed as Hirsutism.

Excessive secretion of male hormone also causes oily skin and acne.

Ovulation mirrors regular periods and anovulation mirrors irregular periods.

Continuous non-formation of egg and therefore absence of progesterone poses a risk of endometrial cancer. (Cancer of the body of the uterus)

We all know that "Insulin" is a hormone that keeps our blood sugar levels under control. Any disturbance in the insulin causes Diabetes. In PCOS there is "Insulin Resistance". Even though the insulin levels are normal, our body doesn't respond to it and that causes our body to secrete more insulin in an attempt to correct the problem. This leads to Hyperinsulenemia and eventually Type II diabetes sets in.

But what causes our body to behave in such a weird manner? Well, there are many reasons given. In 20–40% of cases it runs in families. Obesity, sedentary lifestyle, bad eating habits and stress are all linked with increased risk of PCOS.

Juggling is not only about acne, erratic periods or subfertility. It's also about the mood swings, depression and sleep apnea she keeps fighting with. Many of these symptoms we know about and many we don't understand how they occur. All we can offer is a sympathetic attitude and proper counseling.

So changing lifestyle becomes an important part of managing PCOS and allowing our body to juggle with the hormones effectively.

Chapter 11

Know your Symptoms

Dr. Vimee Bindra

"We should not give up and we should not allow the problem to defeat us."
A P J Abdul Kalam

Know your symptoms !

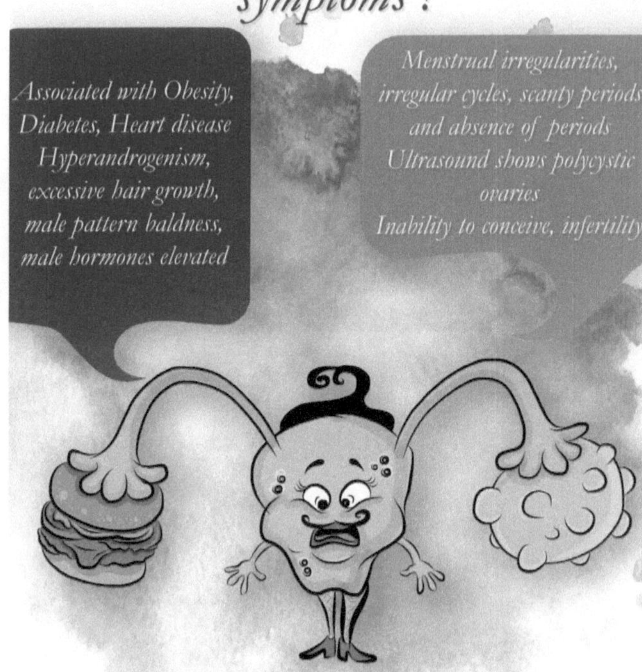

You cannot see what you don't know. So knowing your symptoms is very important for early identification and treatment.

Awareness is the key and identification of the symptoms can save you from long-term consequences of PCOS. Early detection and treatment will help all women with PCOS to keep it suppressed. All women may not have all the symptoms. Some women may have a combination of two three symptoms as well.

Common symptoms of PCOS are

Irregular periods – you may have irregular periods or absence of periods. Women with PCOS may not get their period for two to three months altogether or they may not get it without medication.

Scanty periods – periods may be regular or irregular with reduced flow of blood

Excessive hair growth especially on face, back, chest, chin and inner thighs.

Hair fall especially male pattern baldness, losing scalp hairs and thinning of hairs.

Acne on face and back due to increased androgens (male hormones).

Weight gain and inability to lose weight in spite of exercise and diet.

Fertility problems; many women discover they have PCOS when they are planning to conceive but are unable to do so. In a normal menstrual cycle, women release one egg and if there is no pregnancy, the endometrium sheds down and periods happen. But in PCOS there is no ovulation or delayed ovulation so women don't conceive and find it difficult to become pregnant.

Mood swings, anxiety and depression are also some of the very common signs which are usually recognized by others; especially husbands or close friends notice the change in their behavior.

There are many associated risk with PCOS with diabetes, metabolic syndrome, sleep apnea, stroke and cardiovascular risk; these have been discussed in detail in the respective chapters.

Chapter 12

Lifestyle Management

Dr. Vimee Bindra

"You are essentially who you create yourself to be and all that occurs in your life is the result of your own making."
Stephen Richards

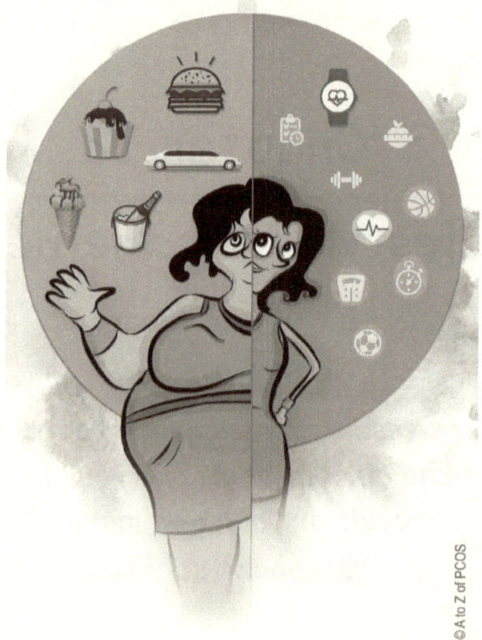

Healthy lifestyle and exercise are an investment for better health in future.

Whenever she visits the doctor, she hears only one thing, do exercise and change your lifestyle. You must be tired of listening this from your doctor but yes believe it or not this is the best treatment for PCOS. If this is followed properly you hardly need to visit a doctor.

Lifestyle Factors that Cause PCOS

There are various factors that contribute to PCOS and dysfunctional follicles. These include stress (leading to the production of high cortisol levels by the adrenal glands), lack of exercise, and poor nutrition. Stress alone can cause anovulatory cycles. Birth control pills shut down normal ovary function, and sometimes it never recovers when the pills are stopped. Our diets are full of petrochemical contaminants also xenobiotics, that derail normal metabolism. We take prescription drugs that impair the functioning of our brain (hypothalamus), which may affect the menstrual cycle.

The average levels of testosterone and androstenedione in obese PCOS women are significantly higher than those in non-obese PCOS women. Women with PCOS are typically prone to high blood sugar, falling into a pre-diabetic range. PCOS disappears rapidly in most women when they cut sugar and refined carbohydrates from their diet.

Lifestyle Changes: Activity Level and What You Eat

If you have PCOS and are overweight, weight loss is the most effective method of restoring normal ovulation and menstruation. As a first step, your doctor may recommend weight loss through a low-calorie diet combined with moderate exercise activities. Using a combined approach of diet and weight loss is important and losing even 5–10% of your total body weight makes a significant impact.

Exercise helps lower blood sugar levels. If you have PCOS, increasing your daily activity and participating in a regular exercise program may treat or even prevent insulin resistance and help you keep your weight under control.

Weight loss: Weight and weight loss can be frustrating. High insulin levels lead to more fat being stored leading to further weight gain and insulin resistance; it's a difficult cycle to break. The other problem is that insulin resistance makes it really difficult to lose weight, even though weight loss will help with insulin resistance. Weight loss reduces the high insulin levels that occur and results in reduction in testosterone levels. A 10 percent loss in body weight can restore a normal period and make your cycle more regular. In addition to improving the chance of regular ovulatory cycles, it may help reduce hair growth and acne. The increased risk of long-term problems such as diabetes, high blood pressure and heart disease are reduced. Even a modest reduction in your weight; for instance, losing 5 percent of your body weight might improve your condition.

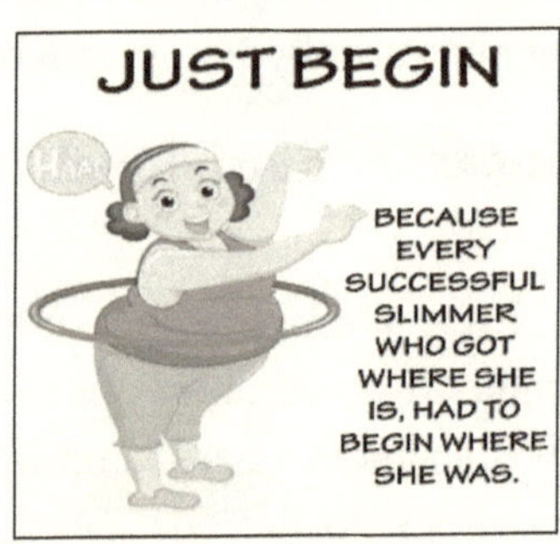

Eating right: Healthy eating tips include:

- Limiting processed foods and foods with added sugars
- Adding more whole-grain products, fruits, vegetables, and lean meats to your diet

Consider how you eat on a daily basis. The best is low glycemic index lifestyles that will help you keep blood sugar levels regulated, possibly lose weight, and for some, help regulate cycles and ovulate. It's important to eat throughout the day for sugar balance; every three hours. Avoid fad diets. Counting calories and fat is not what you need. A balanced diet with whole foods that your body can process and break down in a healthy way is what's most important. Healthy eating can also keep your heart healthy and lower your risk of developing diabetes.

Exercise:

Young women with PCOS often have high levels of insulin. Having high levels of insulin tells your body to store fat and may contribute to PCOS symptoms. Exercise is the only way your body can move sugar from the blood stream into the muscles without insulin. This helps lower insulin levels. Exercise also improves the body's sensitivity to insulin. This means that pancreas doesn't need to produce as much insulin to manage your blood sugar levels. With insulin levels within more normal levels, you should have less of the male hormones in your body and less fat storage, leading to weight loss and return of a more regular cycle. Regular activity can also help improve your mood and boost your energy. If you aren't active now, build up slowly. Work towards moving for at least 60 minutes every day.

Weight Management Tips:

- Start by detoxing – go for the Detox water concoction (prepare 1 litre of water with lemon, cucumber slices and grated ginger and mint leaves, add more colour by adding various berries/ oranges/ fruits to it, leave it overnight in the fridge), drink this daily
- Choose nutritious, high-fibre carbohydrates instead of sugary or refined carbohydrates
- Balance carbohydrates with protein and healthy fats
- Eat small meals and snacks throughout the day instead of large meals
- Exercise regularly to help manage insulin levels and your weight (at least 3 days a week – start with 15 minutes of cardio and while the heart rate is up, start cross-fit training, this helps burn more fat; induce endurance exercises in your regime through yoga/ pilates to ensure enough stretching of muscles)
- Rest for no longer than half hour after a work-out; remember the idea is to be on the move throughout the day in order to keep that metabolism running well.
- Hydrate yourself well; at least 2.5 – 3 Liters of fluids a day (mostly water), avoid coffee in that count. Hydrating well helps eliminate toxin build-up that contributes to weight gain

- Ensure you are enriching yourself with good probiotic supplements/ diet to maintain a good gut flora – WE ARE WHAT WE EAT!

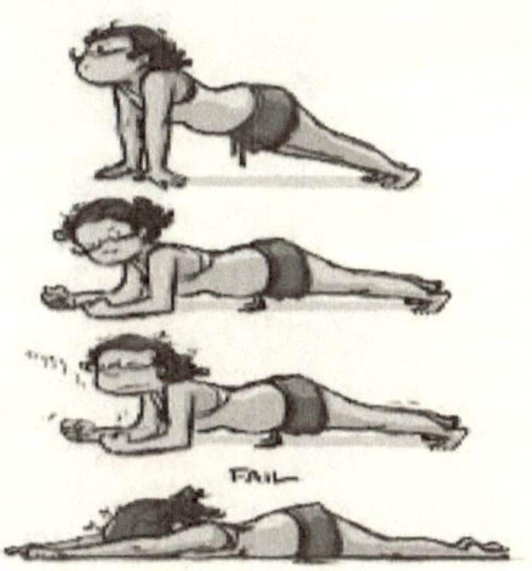

- Stay motivated – join a gym – get a personal trainer if you have to to help you kick start your journey to the **New You**!

Chapter 13

Metformin in PCOS

Dr. R N Mehrotra

"Its your road, and yours alone. Others may walk it with you, but no one can walk it for you..."

Rumi

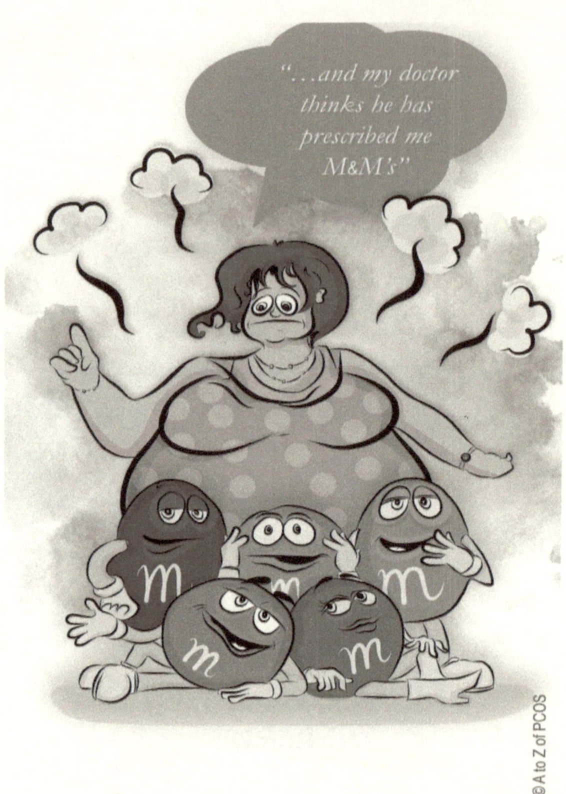

Metformin is a commonly prescribed drug in PCOS. It has some side effects but in few cases its worth it to go through those side effects and wait for the outcome it provides at the end. But it is also over-prescribed so unnecessary usage should be avoided.

Is my doctor treating me or trying to make me sicker by prescribing this medicine? How was your first week on Metformin? Terrible? Filled with bloating, nausea and a sickening feeling? Here's my experience with Metformin

I went to the doctor when I was trying to conceive and was suffering from PCOS two years back. Unfortunately, I went to her one day before I had to attend a wedding and guess what she prescribed me, a drug called Metformin and told me that it also enhances the effect of clomiphene which i am using for fertility treatment. I discussed a few things with her, grabbed my tablets from the pharmacy and started the same day. I could not believe what I was going through, without even eating the wedding food, I was bloated, nauseated and going to the loo every half hour. Was that doctor envious of my social plans??

PCOS- Use of Metformin

The exact reason of PCOS is not known, but many scientists believe that these women are suffering from some kind of insulin resistance at the level of muscles and fatty tissue. Insulin normally acts on these cells, and activates the metabolic machinery which lowers the blood glucose. That means if tissues are resistant to actions of insulin, the pancreas has to produce more Insulin to keep the blood glucose in control. The ovaries are not insulin resistant; therefore they become affected by the increasing insulin levels. Ovaries start producing more of male hormones, and less of good quality eggs which are essential for fertility. The insulin resistance also makes them more vulnerable for developing Diabetes, Fatly liver, lipid abnormalities and heart disease.

Key to successful treatment of PCOS is addressing this insulin resistance. The most important intervention is changes in lifestyle. Aggressive dietary modifications with regular exercise are most important. Many studies have shown the efficacy of lifestyle modifications having a beneficial effect on all manifestations of PCOS.

What is Metformin?

Metformin was first described in 1922 by Emil Werner. French Diabetologist Jean Sterne was the first scientist to evaluate effects of Metformin in treating diabetes and named it Glucophage, "glucose eater". Metformin is known to decrease the glucose production by the liver. It is known to activate a very important enzyme AMP-activated protein kinase, which plays a role in insulin signaling in insulin sensitive tissues. Thus making insulin more effective by decreasing the insulin resistance. Therefore the insulin levels will decline, and would result in improvement in some of the manifestation of PCOS. But it is important to remember that lifestyle changes are more superior to Metformin. Metformin with diet and exercise will give better results.

How Metformin works?
- It reduces hepatic glucose production and intestinal absorption
- It increases peripheral glucose uptake
- Increases SHBG – which in turn reduces androgen levels

Role of Metformin in PCOS
- Especially is used if PCOS women have evidence of glucose metabolism abnormalities like

IGT (Impaired Glucose Tolerance) or IFG.

- It is effective in PCOS women with normal glucose levels also. It can help to ameliorate the cutaneous manifestations of Insulin resistance like skin tags and acanthosis nigricans.
- As stated earlier for obesity, the lifestyle changes are most important, but if the results are not encouraging, metformin can be used.
- Metformin has a beneficial effect in making cycles more regular. It also helps to reduce the androgen levels, though contraceptive pills may be more effective.
- For fertility, clomiphene has been found to be more effective. Metformin alone is not very effective, but improve your chances of fertility in combination with clomiphene.

Side effects of Metformin

Metform in is quite safe; the chances of hypoglycemia are rare. Commonly reported side effects are

- Nausea
- Bloating
- Diarrhoea and metallic taste.

A majority of patients tolerate it quite well. Before initiating metformin it is important to check renal function. Metformin should be initiated slowly and increased to maximum dosage gradually over few weeks.

Tips to avoid Metformin Side effects

- Take the Metformin dose at night time if daily single dose, as you will spend worst of its time while sleeping
- If side effects are really awful, talk to your doctor, she may decrease the dosage for a few weeks till your body gets used to it

- You will get better, you won't be sick everyday and Metformin helps, don't get disappointed.

It is important to remember that there is no single drug for all the manifestations of PCOS. Lifestyle changes are a must; later your Doctor would discuss with you the other options depending on what is your most significant complaint.

My initial few months on Metformin were very tough. I felt I was permanently pregnant as I always had morning sickness. But I kept taking the medication and believe me, things improved and I was free of side effects and above all, I conceived. I am still using Metformin, I rarely have any side effects. My skin changes have become better; I shave my legs less often since I am using Metformin. So my doctor was right but I would advise you not to start Metformin at least one day prior to any social event, function or meeting.

Chapter 14

Nutrition in PCOS

Dr. Deepa Agarwal

"Motivation is what gets you started and Habit is what keeps you going."
Jim Ryun

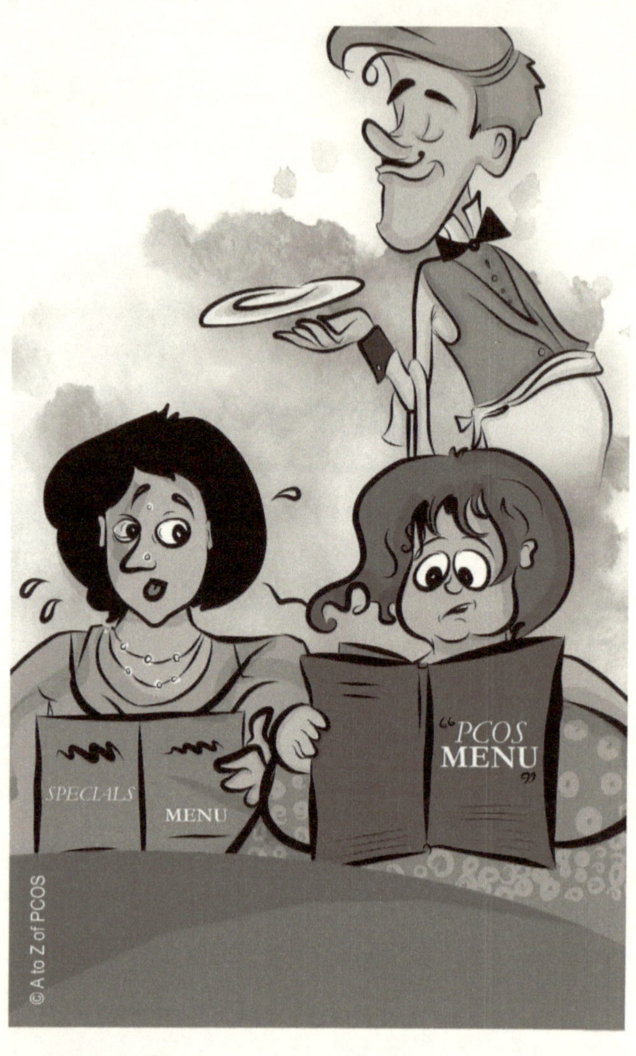

Type of Food You Eat Is Most Important to Keep Your PCOS Under Control

Is this You?

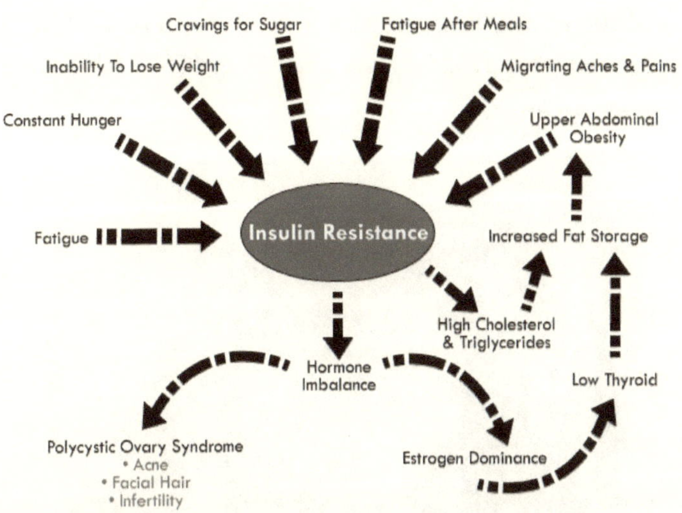

Nutrition in PCOS

Tips for maintaining a healthy weight with PCOS

Polycystic Ovary Syndrome (PCOS) is a condition that affects 5–10% of women of childbearing age. PCOS is associated with: irregular menstrual cycles, abnormal hair growth or loss, abdominal obesity, elevated insulin levels, elevated testosterone levels, polycystic ovaries, dark patches of velvety skin on neck, arms, breasts or thighs, acne, and infertility. Nearly 50% of women with PCOS are overweight or obese. Improving your diet and exercise program by making lifestyle changes may reduce the risk of developing chronic diseases associated with PCOS such as diabetes, heart disease and endometrial cancer. The good news is that losing anywhere from 5 to 10 percent of your body weight can help with weight-related health problems.

The best eating plan if you have PCOS is one that helps you manage your weight and also lower the long-term risks of diabetes and heart disease. This plan should be low in saturated fat and high in fibre. Start by making healthy food choices following the Healthy Eating Plate.

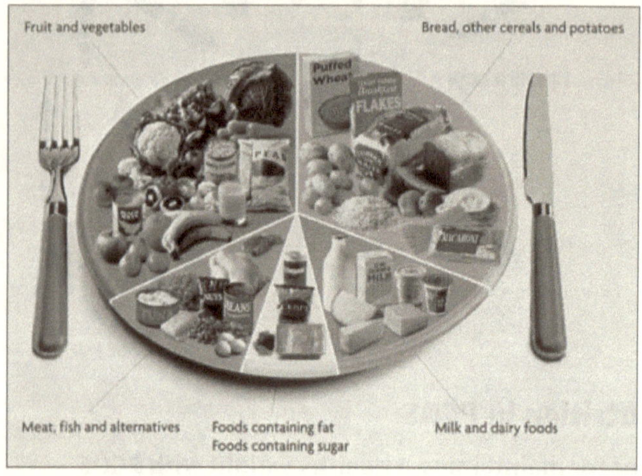

Choose better fats

Too much saturated and trans fat in the diet can lead to weight gain, high blood pressure and high cholesterol. Limit foods that contain saturated and trans fats. Instead of these bad fats, choose smaller amounts of healthy unsaturated fats, which are found in vegetable oils like canola and olive oil, avocado and nuts. Aim for a total of 30 to 45ml (2 to 3 Tbsp) of healthy fats each day.

Increase Fibre

Eating more fibre can help maintain blood sugar levels and lower your cholesterol. Plus, fibre helps make you feel full, so you tend to eat less. This can help with weight control. Aim for 21 to 25 grams per day. Here are some high fibre foods to try:

- Fruit – especially berries, pears, oranges, figs, kiwi, apple, melons
- Vegetables – especially peas, spinach, cauliflower, carrot, gourds etc
- Whole grains – such as oats, brown rice, whole wheat, quinoa, barley, jowar and foxtail millet and buckwheat
- Legumes – such as lentils, chickpeas, soybeans and kidney beans
- Cereals made with wheat bran, psyllium or whole grain oats
- Nuts and seeds – such as almonds, walnuts, flax, sunflower seeds

Enjoy Protein

Similar to fibre, protein also helps you feel full for longer, so you will eat less. This is a great way to help control your weight. Make sure that you have some protein at every meal and snack like chicken, fish or prawns. Bake, grill, broil, boil, steam and microwave foods instead of frying them. Try vegetarian options such as legumes, soy or a quarter cup of nuts or seeds. Milk, low fat yogurt and paneer are also good sources of protein.

Limit salt intake (aim for less than 2400 milligrams of salt per day)

- Use lemon juice, mustard, vinegar, pepper, herbs and spices instead of table salt to season foods.
- Limit foods such as cured and smoked meats, salted nuts, canned and processed vegetables, meats, marinades and sauces.
- Minimize intake of processed foods.

Other Foods to Limit

Some foods cause weight gain if you eat them often. Choose fewer foods that are high in sugar, salt, refined flour and fat such as:

- White Bread, Noodles, Pasta
- Bakery Products like cakes, cookies, biscuits
- Regular soda, malted beverages
- Candy and chocolate and ice cream
- Salty and fried snacks, junk foods, packaged foods

Be Active

Try to get at least 2 ½ hours of exercise each week. Start with 10 minutes of activity and work up to longer times as your body adjusts. Even if you don't lose weight, exercise can help control your blood sugar and cholesterol levels and lower your risk for heart disease and diabetes.

Bottom Line

There is no specific diet that can prevent or treat PCOS. However, eating well and being active can help manage some of the long-term complications of PCOS. An eating plan that is high in fibre and low in saturated and trans fat can help lower the risk of heart disease and diabetes.

PCOS: Hunter-Gatherer Diet

Meat & Fish

Fruits & Berries

Vegetables

Nuts

A hunter-gatherer diet is often the best type of diet for PCOS. This diet is high in healthy proteins such as lean meats, seafood, fruits and berries, vegetables, and nuts and low in grains. Most especially of course, the diet should be low in sugar since hunter-gatherer cultures had very low sugar intake overall. This diet would be varied with respect to quantity and calories for differing weight loss or maintenance requirements.

A simple one day hunter-gatherer diet for PCOS variants

Breakfast: Omelette made with onions and spinach.

Snack: Ambrosia (pear, avocado and 1/2 unripe banana – blend in blender until smooth and creamy)

Lunch: Fish drizzled with olive oil, with brocolli or salad (dressing of fresh lemon, olive oil and fresh herbs)

Snack: Sliced baby cucumber with fresh lemon squeezed on top. 3 tbsp almonds and 1 cup of fresh blueberries

Dinner: Grilled chicken breast with pesto.

Sample Nutrition Plan

Early Morning (6–7am)

Skimmed Milk Tea/ Green Tea- 200ml

Breakfast (8–9am)

2 Chapatis with 1cup Veg Curry

Veg Upma/Poha/Broken Wheat Upma- 1 cup

Sprouts/Plain/Ragi Idlis/Jowar Idlis- 3no.+ 1 cup sambar

Dosas/Wheat panckaes/Moong Dhal pancakes/Besan pancakes- 2 no. + mint chutney

Mid Morning (11–12 noon)

Fruit–1 cup/ Veg.Salad–1cup/ Buttermilk- 200ml/Yogurt – 1 cup/ Nuts (almonds (4–6no.) + Walnuts (4no.))

Lunch (1–2pm)

Brown Rice/ Foxtail Millet/Quinoa- 1 cup/ 2 Plain Chapatis+ 1 cup Veg + 1 cup pulses + 1 cup Curd (Avoid papads, pickles)

Tea time (4–5pm)

Skimmed Milk Tea/ Green Tea- 200ml + Sprouts/Corn Salad- 1cup

Dinner (8pm): Phulkas- 2no. + 1 cup Veg curry or, same as Breakfast

Bed Time- Low fat Milk- 200ml

(Non-Veg: Chicken/Fish- Twice a week, 200g/serving, not fried)

(Egg White (Boiled: 2no. /day))

Chapter 15

Obese and Lean PCOS

Dr. Amita Dhakad, Dr. Vimee Bindra

"Take care of your body. It's the only place you have to live."
Jim Rohn

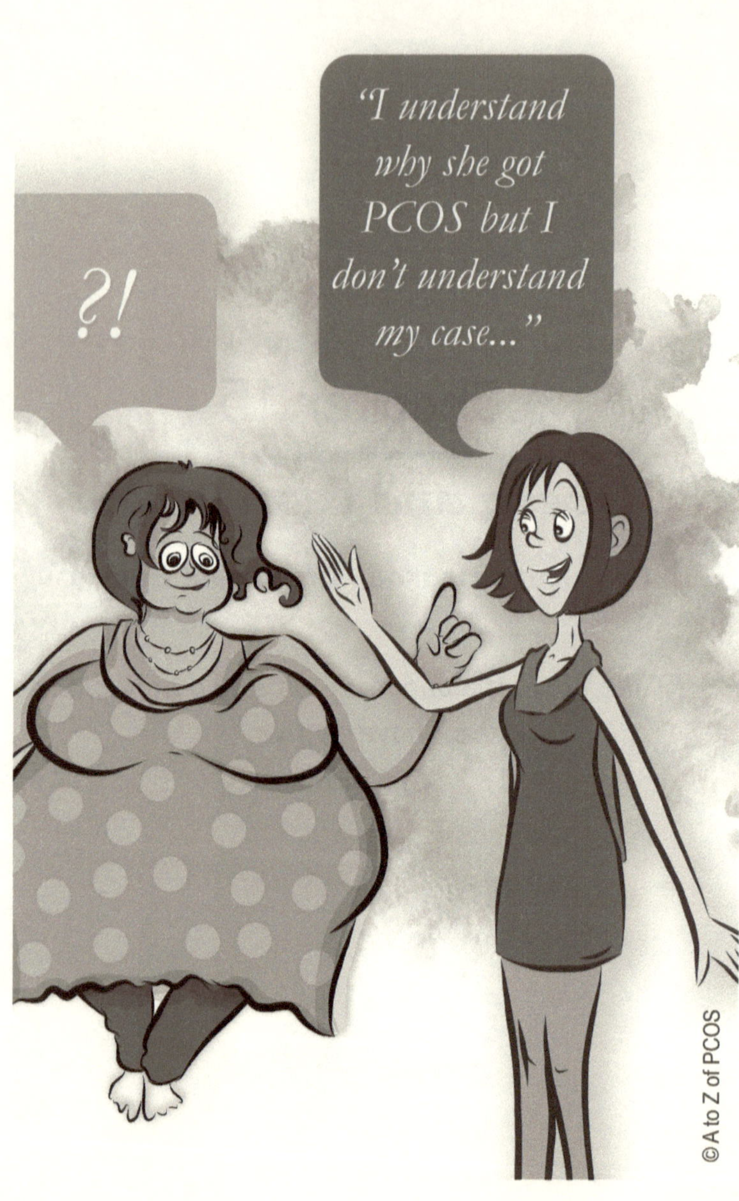
?!
'I understand why she got PCOS but I don't understand my case..."
©A to Z of PCOS

Maria was both worried and surprised. She went to the doctor yesterday for irregular periods and her doctor told her that she has PCOS. She had some knowledge about PCOS and she knew that it happens in overweight and obese women and they keep on gaining weight along with other symptoms such as irregular cycle, acne, hair growth and infertility. It was expected for her to be surprised when she was diagnosed with PCOS as she was perfectly fine for her weight for her height. She had a perfect BMI of 22, then why did she get PCOS? She could not understand and started researching more about it.

Many people think that people who have PCOS are overweight, but this is a myth. In fact, many women with PCOS have normal weight or are underweight. Women with lean PCOS is a group which many people are not even aware of.

There are two main types of PCOS

1. Obese PCOS – A majority of PCOS women (80%) are overweight, high BMI, insulin resistance and typical PCOS symptoms of irregular cycles, ovarian cysts, hair growth, and acne. They are mostly diagnosed when they start trying for pregnancy.

2. Lean PCOS – Some women with PCOS have normal weight or low BMI with or without insulin resistance and exhibit some symptoms such as acne, irregular cycles.

The most common prescription for PCOS women is diet and exercise to lose weight. So what about these 20% of the women? How do they manage their PCOS? This condition is still baffling the patients and doctors as well.

It was found that more than their BMI or overall weight, the type of their body shape was more important and that is determined by the amount of fat in various areas. The fat distribution in majority of these lean PCOS is either android or intermediate types, which means that they have more fat in their upper body under the influence of male hormones as compared to their normal counterparts of equal weight and BMI. Even their visceral fat is more than the normal women of their age. And recent researchers consider this android fat distribution as a surrogate marker for reduced reproductive capability of the woman.

Insulin resistance seems to play an important role in causation of PCOS but it's debatable that lean PCOS suffer from same degree of insulin resistance which is intrinsic but obese PCOS have an additional superimposed IR which may be due to obesity. In several studies it has been seen that the insulin levels are either higher or normal in lean PCOS as compared to obese PCOS but lean PCOS ovaries are very sensitive to insulin as compared to women who do not suffer from PCOS.

Lean or obese PCOS, they share similar risk factors such as cardiovascular disease and other risks associated with PCOS irrespective of body weight with the only difference being the severity and time when it presents. So all women with PCOS irrespective of their body weight should work towards preventing cardiovascular and other health problems. They should be encouraged to be active and keep their food intake towards low glycemic index foods rich in proteins.

Lean PCOS need not lose weight but they need to develop better eating habits and an exercise regimen which would not cause weight gain. Eat more vegetables, fruits, healthy gluten free food.

If you are a lean PCOS, you are doing pretty well. You just need to be aware of it. Do exercise, maintain your BMI and have a healthy eating habit.

Chapter 16

Pregnancy with PCOS

Dr. Pooja Sharma Dimri

"Life is not about finding yourself. Life is about creating yourself"
Lolly Daskal

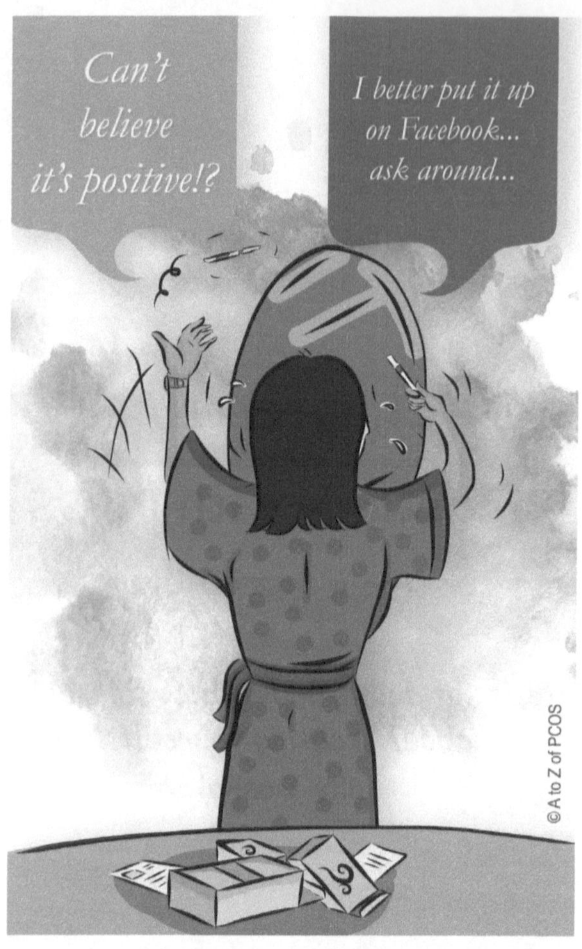

PCOS women with irregular periods who are trying for pregnancy are so habituated to get negative pregnancy test results that they really can't believe when their tests come out as positive and they keep showing their tests to other women for confirmation. And they keep on doing the test several times just to make themselves believe....

keerti suffered from severe PCOS and she shares what she underwent through the years when she was trying for pregnancy.

"Late pregnancy scares many of us, especially when you are in your thirty plus. We not only become a victim of scrutiny but you also scrutinize every occurrence in your sex life. You not only go through mental trauma but emotionally you shatter yourself and either you take charge of it or start playing a blame game. A life in us is not by will of two bodies but by the will of God and God alone.

I am Keerti, a thirty six year old and a PCOS patient. It's so important for any women getting married in their late 20's or 30's that when they are planning for child, they should consult a doctor and discuss the same. Well I did the same and when I was thirty three years old, I went for a routine check-up. I had undergone two IUI'S and nothing happened. This was an early sign that I should have come earlier to get myself checked but I went through a trauma. I broke down many times but I haven't given up on God's work. I quit my work eventually just to conceive (cause of my age factor). I then decided to change my doctor and kept reading a lot on the internet.

Finally I met an amazing and blessed doctor. In one of my first conversations, she instilled an immense hope saying that children are the gift of God and that doctors are the instruments God uses to help patients. Wow! This is what made me stick around and my journey begins from there.

I was regularly checked for three months and took shots but nothing happened. That's when the doctor asked me to undergo few check-ups. I had undergone an HSG Check-up where they check if your fallopian tube is blocked. It's a bit painful but it was good to know that all was clear.

That's when the doctor decided that she needed to look inside and suggested to undergo laparoscopy. By doing this we were trying to rule out the possibility of anything being wrong. Finally, the day had come and before I went to the operation theatre, the doctor had come to see me and I did mention how nervous I was and how glad I was that she had come and met me with a strong sense of hope. When I woke up it felt as if it all had happened in 10 minutes. I had cyst and everything was alright except that they put some pores on my ovaries. I got discharged the same evening. I remembered my mum being so scared and asking me not to go through this surgery. But I wanted to find out and I am glad now as I hold a healthy 8 month old in my arms and he is adorable. While I was out of surgery, I decided to wait and get things normal inside of me and my periods were still irregular but I didn't bother too much about it. I needed much change in me.

Post surgery and after almost a year, I checked my pregnancy. We were more than seven weeks. But the joy you get when you see the two lines is unimaginable. My husband cried more than me. We thanked God and prayed for this child. But I would tip my hat to the optimistic approach that my doctor had throughout."

PCOS (Polycystic Ovarian Syndrome) is a very common condition affecting women of reproductive age. The prevalence of this disease is increasing day by day. As high as 1 in 10 women are suffering from this condition worldwide. As in PCOS, there is a problem of ovulation or egg production, so conceiving may be a challenge. It is an important cause of infertility. But with lifestyle changes and drugs for ovulation, women with PCOS can conceive and have healthy babies.

Pregnancy in women with PCOS may be considered high risk as compared to the general population. There is a higher risk of miscarriage or abortion linked to PCOS may be as high as such pregnancies are three times the normal risk.

Women suffering from PCOS may be at higher risk of medical problems in pregnancy. These are gestational diabetes mellitus (pregnancy induced), heart disease and preeclampsia (high blood pressure in pregnancy). There is also a high risk of prenatal and post-natal depression. These antenatal patients are more likely to require caesarean section or operative delivery. The babies of these women are more likely to be born preterm and kept in neonatal intensive care units.

A woman with PCOS may have difficulty in conceiving and may require medication in the form of ovulation induction to conceive. Once she conceives, she is very anxious about the pregnancy. One of the patients Ritu, a thirty two year old was trying to get pregnant for the past 8 years. She was a known case of PCOS since she was nineteen and was on medication for irregular periods. After she failed to conceive naturally, she was put on drugs for ovulation induction as there is an aberrant ovulation in these patients. She conceived 2 years back but had a spontaneous abortion at the 7th week of pregnancy. She was dejected and depressed. With treatment, she conceived again and came to me for advice. She was worried about the outcome of this pregnancy. You will find many patients like her who suffering from PCOS, conceive after a long frustrating treatment and then face a risk of complications during pregnancy. So what is the way forward?

Your Doctor is your Best Friend!

If you are expecting, with a background of PCOS, you should be under care of an experienced obstetrician. As soon as you conceive, meet your doctor to outline a plan of management for the duration of pregnancy. You should understand how PCOS affects the outcome of pregnancy at different times. You should be aware of what complications to expect and how to deal with them. Also, PCOS is a harbinger of many medical problems like diabetes, so one should be ready to prevent and tackle the consequences.

Diet and Weight Gain

You should work with your obstetrician and dietician to work out a diet plan for pregnancy based on your body mass index (BMI). Gaining the right amount of weight is absolutely essential to reduce pregnancy complications especially if you are overweight or obese. The importance of eating well and staying active cannot be overemphasized. Your diet plan for pregnancy should be under the supervision of a nutritionist. But I will just mention the general guidelines. Avoid too much of trans fat and saturated fats. Instead use healthy unsaturated fats in the cooking. Eat a high fibre diet which includes fruits, vegetables, whole grains and pulses. This maintains blood sugar levels and prevents excessive weight gain. High fibre diet also avoids constipation which is very common during pregnancy. During pregnancy, you also need a high intake of protein which is essential for the baby's growth and development. As for protein rich foods that you can consume during pregnancy are pulses, legumes and soy for vegetarians along with milk and milk products like curd and paneer. The other good sources of proteins are chicken, fish and egg whites. It is better to cook the protein in less amount of fat and bake or grill instead of deep frying. It is better to avoid excess salt in diet like pickles, papad, spraying on salad etc. Take small, frequent meals.

Antenatal Check-ups

You should be regular in your pregnancy check-ups as advised by your doctor. Your doctor will advise investigations and sonography as required. In your case, the frequency of visits may be more than a low risk pregnant lady. Be sure to take all the medicines and supplements as advised. Ask your doctor about any warning signals or signs of any complications.

Delivery

As discussed earlier, because of the high incidence of pregnancy-induced hypertension, gestational diabetes and preterm labor, there is a higher chance of baby being born preterm and requiring neonatal intensive care. Also you may have higher chances of ending up with a C-section. Therefore, plan your delivery in a higher setup where all the facilities are available along with a neonatologist to take care of your baby.

To conclude, PCOS with pregnancy needs special attention and care. Proper planning, advice and regular monitoring under supervision of the obstetrician will lead to a successful pregnancy with a healthy mother and baby.

Few Tips Shared by Keerti for PCOS Cysters

1. Be happy, eat healthy and stay healthy.

2. Do what you love to do but at any point do not release worry/stress hormones (the eggs cannot take too much of stress) instead be happy and happy hormones helps us to conceive.

3. Your pregnancy is your own and no one else's business. So don't get depressed by hearing to your elders or when you see a baby or any women carrying her baby. Instead imagine yourself carrying a baby always.

4. Follow every check-up and medicines.

5. Don't be too anxious. Just relax during your ovulation and make sure you and partner come together.

6. Be careful and make sure at least post ovulation you take no stress and take good amount of rest. And get foot massages if possible.

7. Stay positive, and meditate.

Chapter 17

Quotient of Life with PCOS

Dr. Seema Pandey

"Be thankful for what you have; you'll end up having more. If you concentrate on what you don't have, you will never, ever have enough"
Oprah Winfrey

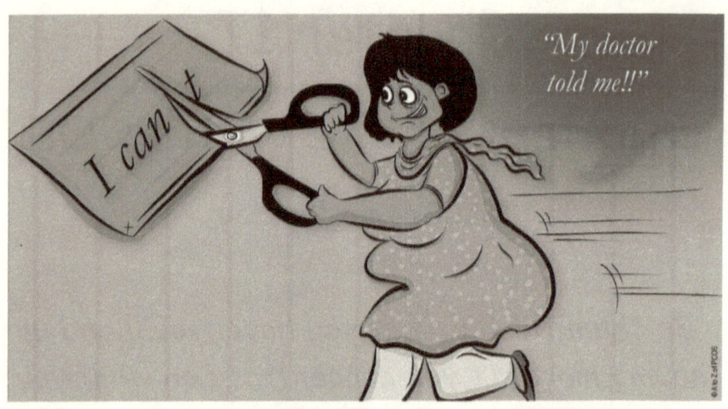

PCOS can be controlled and it is you who can control it and live a healthy and happy life

The psychological implications of PCOS are easily underestimated and have been largely ignored. The impact is as great as smooth hairless bodies and faces, regular menstruation and the capacity to bear children were thought to be classic feminine traits and as a result of their symptoms, PCOS ladies express their feelings of being different from others and being less feminine. And that's why PCOS was taken as a deeply stigmatizing condition or as a thief of womanhood.

As there is currently no cure , the management of PCOS is directed towards improving the patients' health related quality of life(HRQoL) by means of symptomatic alleviation and prevention of long-term complications including development of the metabolic syndrome and associated sequels(such as diabetes mellitus and heart ailment).

HPQoL is defined as multidimensional concept that encompasses physical, emotional and social aspects associated with a specific disease or its treatment. So HPQoL measurement gives important information on the benefits of medical treatment or interventions from the patient's perspective. Prior research has suggested that PCOS and its associated symptomatic profile have a negative impact on quality of life.

A few days back, I met my colleague and she was really disturbed as her eighteen year old daughter was behaving strangely. She was a lively girl who used to enjoy life and the company of new people and then all of sudden she went into seclusion. On further probing the mother I came to know that for the last one year, her periods were irregular and used to stop only on medications. She was putting on weight and her face especially the lower jaw area was full of hair. As long as the hairy areas (limbs) were hidden, she was not bothered about it. But now she started feeling ashamed of her body image. When I examined her I diagnosed PCOS and her androgens (male hormones) were found to be very high. She started crying in front of me as she was not able to face the piercing eyes of her peers and friends. While talking about the options she was totally against waxing (local treatment) of these hairy areas as she found it very painful. All she wanted was a quick miraculous treatment so that all her symptoms could disappear. That is a typical behavior shown by young girls suffering from PCOS. Altered self perception, fear of impaired sexual functioning and problems at work place are few other problems these women face. Once they plan to have a baby, the subfertility and menstrual irregularity brings tension within the family. Many mothers-in-laws come to visit me and suggest correcting the menstrual cycles of their daughters-in-laws. This is so because one can conceive only when the periods are regular. For that farfetched dream they keep changing their doctors and ultimately only get more depressed.

The key is finding someone who can explain the disease in their own language along with the short-term and long term-goals like changing the life style, control of weight, keeping hormonal balance and then planning a family. Once these woman start knowing themselves their agony decreases and then they follow what we the clinicians suggest.

Chapter 18

Relationship Between Hypothyroidism and Hyperprolactinemia With PCOS

Dr. Asha Reddy

"Turn your wounds into wisdom"
Oprah Winfrey

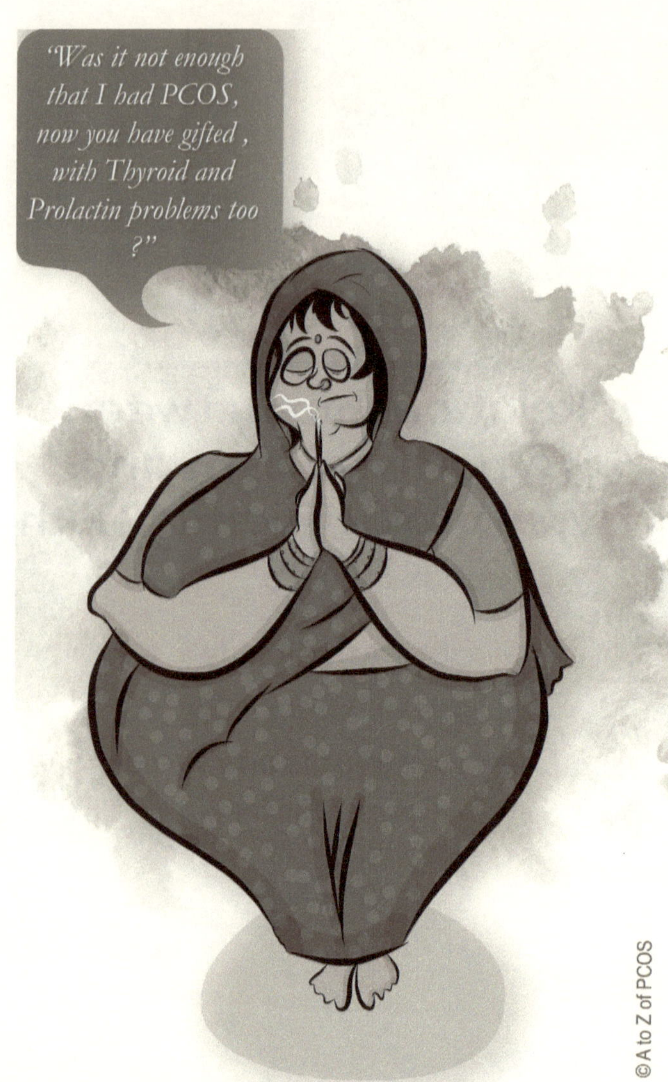
'Was it not enough that I had PCOS, now you have gifted , with Thyroid and Prolactin problems too ?"
© A to Z of PCOS

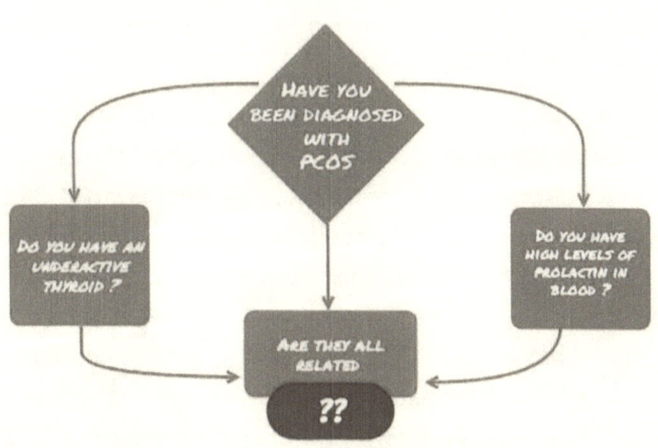

Do you have PCOS (Polycystic Ovarian Syndrome)? Have you been told you have a thyroid disorder? Do you have high prolactin levels? Are PCOS and hypothyroidism related? Are PCOS and hyperprolactinemia related?

Many women with PCOS may also have a thyroid problem, usually hypothyroidism (underactive thyroid) and hyperprolactinemia (high levels of prolactin).

Dr. Stein and Dr. Leventhal first described PCOS in 1935. PCOS affects around 5–15% of the female population. The increasing incidence over the recent years is thought to be related to changing life styles, stress, environmental pollution and endocrine-disruptor-chemicals. Prevalence figures vary depending on the population and diagnostic criteria used.

The cause of this common, poorly understood syndrome is not very certain. PCOS is a combination of polycystic ovaries and disturbed endocrine, reproductive and metabolic disturbances. Women with PCOS commonly present with menstrual disturbances which may include amenorrhea, infertility, acne and or hirsutism. Polycystic ovaries are very common. However, all women with polycystic ovaries do not have the syndrome.

Thyroid disorders and polycystic ovary syndrome (PCOS) are two of the most common hormone problems in women. Thyroid disorders are more common in women with PCOS as compared to the normal population. PCOS is more common in women with hypothyroidism and the symptoms of PCOS can be worse in women who are very overweight. Although hypothyroidism and PCOS are different, the two conditions share many similar features and sometimes women with hypothyroidism may be wrongly diagnosed as having PCOS and vice-versa. Women with PCOS may also have higher levels of prolactin than others. Hypothyroidism can lead to increased prolactin levels in about a third of women with hypothyroidism and these women may have symptoms due to excess prolactin. Both genetic and environmental factors are believed to be contributing to thyroid disorders in PCOS. Whether this is due to some common cause for these disorders or due to a connection among the disorders is not very clear yet. However what is important is that women with PCOS need to be checked for thyroid disturbances as well as altered prolactin levels and treated appropriately.

The thyroid gland is present in the neck region and works as a regulator of various body functions including the rate at which our body converts food for energy, metabolism and other systems. If the thyroid works less this slows the metabolism and results in symptoms such as menstrual irregularities [abnormal bleeding, oligomenorrhea (few periods) or amenorrhea (no periods)] weight gain , anovulation (no ovulation- no release of egg), infertility which are seen in women with PCOS too. Hypothyroidism is known to cause PCOS-like ovaries and overall worsening of PCOS and insulin resistance. Symptoms of hypothyroidism usually appear slowly over several months or years. The lower the thyroid hormone levels, the more severe the symptoms will be.

Other symptoms common to PCOS and hypothyroidism are: blood sugar problems leading to diabetes, high cholesterol levels, and increased testosterone (male hormone) levels leading to acne, scalp hair loss (male pattern baldness), hirsutism (excessive hair growth, male pattern), acanthosis nigricans (darkening of the skin at the nape of the neck and under arms) which is an indicator of hyperinsulinemia and insulin resistance. Insulin resistance, diabetes and obesity aggravate the problem of PCOS.

Dietary excess of sugar creates high insulin levels, which stimulate androgen production in the ovary, which suppresses ovulation. Hypothyroidism can worsen insulin resistance and increase androgen levels. Some reports suggest that hypothyroidism and autoimmune types of thyroid disease are more common in women with PCOS as compared to the normal population.

All cells in the body rely on the hormones secreted from thyroid to function properly. In addition to controlling the rate at which your body converts carbohydrates, protein, and fats into fuel, thyroid hormones also control your heart rate and can affect your menstrual cycle, thus affecting fertility.

To diagnose hypothyroidism, your doctor usually evaluates symptoms, medical history, risk factors, and family history, and then performs a physical exam. Certain blood tests including TSH are necessary. An abnormally high TSH test may mean you have hypothyroidism. Additionally other tests in the thyroid panel (such as Free T4, free T4 index, total T4, T3 and Reverse T3; Thyroid antibodies) and to detect autoimmune thyroid conditions like Hashimoto's may also be necessary. The prolactin levels are measured by a blood test.

Women with PCOS and/or hypothyroidism and hyperprolactinemia have a good reason to avoid sugar and refined carbohydrates such as white bread and pasta. A low fat diet with adequate protein and plenty of vegetables and fibre will often help to restore normal balance. Aerobic or endurance-type exercises are good ways of regulating the insulin levels and associated symptoms. These women may need periodic treatment with progesterones to induce bleeding and correct menstrual irregularities. If there is a low thyroid function (hypothyroid), ovulation and fertility may be restored by supplementing thyroid medication. Ovarian cysts may also resolve. Coexisting Vitamin D deficiency, if present; needs to be treated. Keeping thyroid hormone production in balance requires the right amount of iodine. Too little or too much iodine can cause or worsen hypothyroidism. The main food sources of iodine include dairy products, chicken, beef, pork, fish, and iodized salt. Discuss with your doctor before taking iodine supplements. Appropriate treatment is required to decrease prolactin levels in some women with PCOS. The type of medication necessary is best decided by the treating doctor. Eating excessive amounts of soy and gluten can also affect the thyroid activity. A nutritionist will help in offering additional advice regarding a healthy balanced diet.

Chapter 19

Surgery in PCOS

Dr. Vimee Bindra

"Stop being okay with the norm, seek to transform"
Constance Chuksfriday

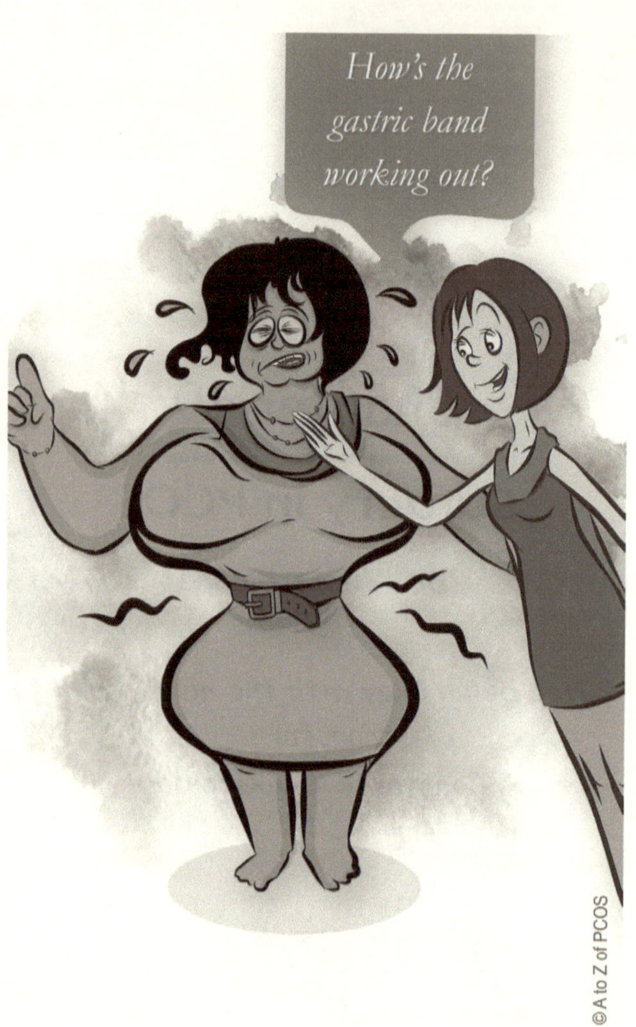

Don't be under the impression that getting your surgery done in the form of ovarian drilling and gastric banding will cure your PCOS.

"I got my surgery done for PCOS, I am free from PCOS now" Is this true? Is surgery the main treatment for PCOS-like other conditions such as fibroids or ovarian cysts? The answer is NO.

Name of this disorder POLYCYCTIC OVARIES leaves an impression that a woman is having multiple cysts in her ovaries and people do believe that it can be cured if the cysts are removed. But my dear Cysters, it's a misnomer as there are no cysts, it's the multiple follicles which are not growing and give an appearance of multiple fluid filled spaces which look like small cysts.

What Is the Role of Surgery in PCOS?

When medications do not work for fertility and regularizing the cycles, you may need to undergo laparoscopic ovarian drilling or waffle ball procedure or modified wedge resection.

What is ovarian drilling and how does it help treating PCOS?

PCOS ovaries have a thick outer layer which produces more testosterone, which results in irregular cycles, acne, hair growth and anovulation and infertility. Ovarian drilling helps breaking that thick layer, draining the fluid collected which helps in decreasing the testosterone levels. This helps woman get her regular period and it helps her conceive also.

How is ovarian drilling done?

Ovarian drilling is done by laparoscopy, a keyhole surgery. A small cut is made at your belly button and a telescope is inserted through it to see your ovaries, and through one or two more small 5mm cuts on either side of abdomen, some extra instruments are inserted and small punctures are made in your ovaries using electrosurgical sources and this helps lower your testosterone levels.

When surgery should be done in PCOS?

- When fertility medicines do not work or ovulation does not happen with higher doses of gonadotropins, then to make ovaries more sensitive to these drugs, drilling may be required to help you ovulate and conceive.
- Drilling should never be done in young adolescent girls with irregular periods or when are just diagnosed PCOS. It should be kept only for cases resistant to ovulation by fertility medications.

What are the advantages of ovarian drilling?

- Ovarian drilling may help women ovulate better and help them conceive. About 50% women may conceive after drilling within one year. Some women may not have regular cycles after drilling.
- Ovarian drilling is a onetime treatment unlike fertility medications which may be required every month. **IT SHOULD NOT BE DONE AGAIN AND AGAIN.**
- For some women, drilling may not fix their problem with regular cycles and ovulation, but it helps fertility medications to work better.

What are the risks involved with ovarian drilling?

- Decision to do drilling should be taken wisely. It should not be done only to regularize cycles if you are not trying to conceive. There are medications available to regularize periods.

- If damage is done to ovarian tissue, this procedure may have adverse effects on future fertility and in some cases may lead to premature menopause.

- Post-procedure, there may be scarring between ovaries and fallopian tubes, which may affect fertility.

Role of bariatric surgery in PCOS

Bariatric surgery can be an effective means of weight loss in PCOS women. Surgical techniques have become safer and less invasive over time and have been found to be effective in achieving significant weight loss. Surgical options have also increased, giving patients more choices. Bariatric surgery may prevent or reverse metabolic syndrome. Bariatric surgery may also have reproductive benefits in PCOS patients. Although bariatric surgery has historically been performed in older, reproductive aged women, it has recently gained favor in adolescents as well. This is of particular importance due to the prevalence of both PCOS and MS (metabolic syndrome) in adolescents. Treatment of PCOS and MS certainly requires a combination of medical therapy, psychological support and lifestyle modifications. These treatments are difficult and often frustrating for patients and physicians. Bariatric surgery can be effective in achieving significant weight loss, restoration of the hypothalamic pituitary axis, reduction of cardiovascular risk and even in improving pregnancy outcomes. Ultimately, bariatric surgery should be considered part of the treatment in PCOS women, especially in those with MS.

The most common methods of bariatric surgery are laparoscopic gastric bypass and laparoscopic adjustable gastric banding (LAGB). Bariatric surgery limits the amount of food the stomach can hold, and/or limits the amount of calories absorbed, by surgically reducing the stomach's capacity to a few ounces.

Bariatric surgery is a powerful tool that should not be overlooked simply because a woman is young or presents with PCOS and MS rather than diabetes mellitus, myocardial infarction and severe chronic hypertension. Although surgery has both short and long term risks, the potential benefits may be greater in these PCOS women than in older women who are already more advanced with respect to vascular disease. Every woman with PCOS and MS deserves to at least be offered education and counseling regarding the role of bariatric surgery in reducing their illness. More importantly, young women undergoing bariatric surgery should be specifically included in research to improve knowledge of long-term outcomes. Bariatric surgery should be considered along with other medical and lifestyle alterations as the first-line therapy in PCOS women with obesity and MS.

Morbidity and mortality in general is inversely proportional to both hospital and surgeon volume. Bariatric surgery is cost effective in comparison to the excessive cost of medical care in these patients for metabolic abnormalities, especially diabetes mellitus In addition to the overwhelming medical evidence for benefits after surgery. Studies also show that patients experience emotional, body image and quality of life improvements after bariatric surgery.

Chapter 20

Treatment for Infertility

Dr. Seema Pandey

*"Nothing is impossible, the word itself says,
I'm possible!"*
Audrey Hepburn

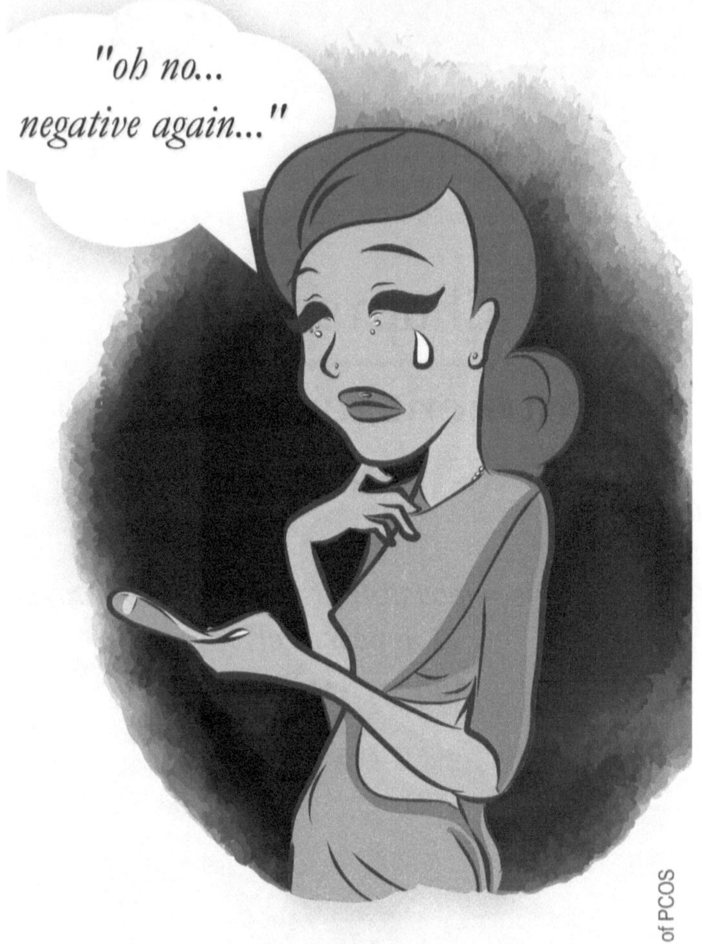

A very common situation faced by women suffering from PCOS.

Whenever I talk to a woman who is diagnosed with PCOS her first question usually is, "Doctor, if I take a course of treatment, will it be cured forever?" And it really takes a while to instill that PCOS is a condition which is not curable unlike typhoid or malaria and will remain in your system but it can be controlled. It's really sad that medical science could not define an optimal cure for infertile women suffering from PCOS. Whenever I start with lifestyle modifications, my client's face becomes tensed as if I am also blaming her for her obesity, her infrequent periods or that I am questioning her intelligence to judge what's good for her. Here I have to take a pause and explain to her that life style modification is not merely eating a low carbohydrate diet or sacrificing her favorite doughnuts. It's more about eating right and living a balanced life. Pharmaceutical agents like clomiphene citrate, insulin sensitizing agents, gonadotropins and GnRH analogues to the use of laparoscopic ovarian drilling and the use of laparoscopic ovarian drilling and the application of assisted reproductive technique.

To sort out these controversies surrounding the treatment of this enigmatic syndrome led to a second meeting of the same group of ESHRE and ASRM held in Thessaloniki, Greece in 2007. They addressed the therapeutic challenges raised in women with efficacy as well as their safety. A panel of experts from across the world was invited to discuss the treatment of women with PCOS and infertility to arrive at a consensus regarding therapy. On the basis of currently available evidence, the following guideline was prepared.

1. Lifestyle modification especially weight reduction and exercise is the first line of treatment.

2. Recommended first line of treatment for ovulation induction remains anti-estrogen clomiphene citrate (CC).
3. Recommended second line intervention should CC fail to result in pregnancy, are either exogenous gonadotropins or laparoscopic ovarian surgery (LOS).
4. Recommended third line treatment is IVF.
5. If a woman say suffers only from PCOS, OI plus TIC (timed intercourse) gives equal result as OI plus IUI.
6. Metformin use in PCOS should be restricted to women with glucose intolerance. Based on recent data available in the literature, the routine use of this drug in OI is not recommended.
7. Insufficient evidence is currently available to recommend the clinical use of aromatase inhibitors for routine ovulation induction.
8. Even singleton pregnancies in PCOS are associated with increased health risk for both the mother and the fetus.

Lifestyle modifications

As I previously mentioned life style modification is not only about losing weight or eating a diet with low carbohydrate. It's all about making yourself ready to bear the child safely so during pre-conception counseling, women are advised to start on folic acid. They are asked to quit smoking and lessen the amount of alcohol they consume.

Weight reduction

The ideal amount of weight loss is unknown, but a 5% decrease of body weight might be clinically meaningful, so women are explained about the positive effects of even losing 5–10% of body weight and how it increases their chances of regular ovulation and thus pregnancy but also the reduction in overall morbidity once they become pregnant (miscarriages and late pregnancy complications). Losing weight is of prime importance to each woman and more to a PCOS lady as the effect of any fertility medication becomes more effective after losing a certain amount, be it CC or gonadotropins or ovarian drilling. So weight loss is recommended as the first-line therapy in obese women with PCOS seeking pregnancy. This recommendation is based on extrapolation from the benefits of weight loss seen in multiple conditions such as diabetes and cardiovascular disease, as well as recognition of obesity's association with poor reproductive outcome. The treatment of obesity is multifaceted and involves behavioral counseling, lifestyle therapy (diet and exercise), pharmacologic treatment, and bariatric surgery. However, there are no perfect studies to guide the choice of such interventions to win over the infertility in women with PCOS. Generally, a combination of medical and behavioral therapies offers the greatest weight loss.

The effects of calorie restriction, increased physical activity, and pharmacologic and weight loss agents in the periconceptional period are unknown and are potentially harmful to our ultimate dream and that is a live healthy baby. These interventions should be conducted before pregnancy, not concurrently with infertility treatment.

Diet

Increasing evidence in women without PCOS suggests that diets with reduced glycemic (carb) load may be beneficial in alleviating hyperinsulinemia and its metabolic consequences. This is of particular importance to women with PCOS because of the close association between insulin resistance and reproductive health. In the absence of level I evidence, the recommended diet for obese women with PCOS is any hypo-caloric diet (with a 500 Kcal/day deficit) with reduced glycemic load and, failing that, any calorie restricted diet with which patients can comply and achieve a 5% weight loss.

Exercise

Several studies have examined combination therapy of diet and exercise. Most of them, however, were not randomized trials, and exercise was not supervised but rather consisted of lifestyle counseling. Although weight loss alone appeared to improve menstrual frequency, the contribution of exercise alone could not be determined in these studies. It is clear that regular physical activity is an important component of weight loss programs because it is associated with better long-term weight loss maintenance. However, its independent role in achieving weight reduction and improved reproductive outcome is less obvious. Increased physical activity is recommended for obese women with PCOS.

But ladies, a word of caution here. Please see your physician before running or involving yourself in any strenuous exercise so that you are safe.

Surgery and medications

The available literature supports the adjuvant use of bariatric surgery and medicinal weight loss for the treatment of obesity in PCOS although large clinical trials are needed. In morbidly obese women, the PCOS phenotype appears to be very frequent and most importantly PCOS has been found to improve markedly after sustained weight loss after bariatric surgery. Anti-obesity drugs have been used in obese women with PCOS although few quality studies have been published. It should be noted that these treatments should not be considered as first-line therapy for obesity in women with PCOS.

Clomiphene citrate

Looking at its cost effectiveness, ease of oral administration with minimal adverse effects reported, minimal ovarian monitoring required and plenty of data regarding its use in PCOS, CC is considered as the first-line medical agent for ovulation induction agent in a PCOS female. Though the exact mechanism of action is not known, CC is said to block the negative feedback mechanisms which results in increased amount of FSH. The main factors that predict the outcome of treatment are obesity, hyperandrogenemia, and age. Ovarian volume and menstrual status also affect the outcome.

- Minimal required dose is 50 mg per day which can be safely raised up to 150 mg a day. The FDA recommended dose is up to 750mg per cycle.

- The overall ovulation rate in PCOS females is 75–80%.

- The overall conception rate per cycle is 22%.

- Multiple pregnancy rate is <10%.

- It should be kept in mind that the duration of treatment should not exceed beyond 6 cycles.

- The drug is usually well tolerated but the common side effects are hot flushes, visual disturbances and headaches.

- OHSS is rare.
- Anti-estrogenic effect on endometrium and cervical mucus is idiosyncratic.

Combination therapy

There is no clear cut evidence of benefit by adding Dexamethasone or Metformin on OI.

Other Anti-estrogens

Tamoxifen is another member of CC family and is said to be as effective as CC for people who cannot tolerate CC.

Aromatase inhibitors

The common ones in use are letrozole and variants like anestrazole. Looking at the paucity of information, it's effectively at par with CC but it is not recommended as first-line therapy.

Insulin Sensitizing Agents

Biguanides and the thiazolidindiones are two main groups of medicines which have been used in diabetic patients and were also used in PCOS women. Metformin is a biguanide and the most commonly used molecule. Pioglitazone and Rosiglitazone are from another group but are not preferred over Metformin because of their safety profile.

With regard to the use of metformin for induction of ovulation, two RCTs have indicated that metformin does not increase live-birth rates above those observed with CC alone in either obese or normal weight women with PCOS. The larger of these two trials demonstrated a selective disadvantage to metformin compared with CC and no apparent advantage to adding metformin to CC, except perhaps in women with BMI >35 kg/m^2 and in those with CC resistance. Results in this trial were the same when subjected to either intention-to-treat analysis or analysis based on adherence: CC resulted in higher ovulation, conception, pregnancy, and live-birth rates compared with metformin, but the combination of both drugs did not result in a significant benefit.

At present, only those women who are having glucose intolerance should take Metformin.

Let your obstetrician decide whether Metformin is to be continued during pregnancy or not.

Metformin alone is less effective than CC in inducing ovulation in women with PCOS.

There seems to be no advantage to adding metformin to CC in women with PCOS.

Gonadotropins and GnRH analogues

These are the hormones which are released by the pituitary gland and hypothalamus in brain and govern the follicular growth in ovaries. These are expensive medications and can have serious side effects and should not be self-administered.

The aim of ovulation induction for women with anovulatory PCOS is to restore fertility and achieve a singleton live pregnancy.

All these medications are to be used under strict monitoring of your fertility specialist.

We use low dose of gonadotropins in women who have failed to ovulate with oral medications like CC and letrozole.

Multiple pregnancies and hyper-stimulation are two of the most dreaded side effects.

Strict cancellation criteria: Your fertility specialist may discuss with you before starting these medications.

The significantly higher hyper-stimulation rate, the associated risk of multiple pregnancies, and the additional inconvenience and cost of concomitant GnRH agonist administration, in the absence of documented increases in pregnancy success, do not currently justify the routine use of GnRH agonists during ovulation induction with gonadotropins in women with PCOS.

Laparoscopic Ovarian Surgery

Surgical approaches to ovulation induction have developed from the traditional wedge resection to modern day minimal access techniques, usually employing laparoscopic ovarian diathermy or laser. Multiple ovarian puncture performed either by diathermy or by laser is known as ovarian drilling. A separate chapter is dedicated to this topic.

- Laparoscopic ovarian surgery can achieve mono-follicular ovulation with no risk of OHSS or high-order multiples.
- Intensive monitoring of follicular development is not required after LOS.
- Laparoscopic ovarian surgery is an alternative to gonadotropin therapy for CC-resistant anovulatory PCOS.
- The treatment is best suited to those for whom frequent ultrasound monitoring is impractical.
- Laparoscopic ovarian surgery is a single treatment using existing equipment.
- The risks of surgery are minimal and include the risks of laparoscopy, adhesion formation, and destruction

of normal ovarian tissue. Minimal damage should be caused to the ovaries. Irrigation with an adhesion barrier may be useful, but there is no evidence of efficacy from prospective studies. Surgery should be performed by appropriately trained personnel.

- Laparoscopic ovarian surgery should not be offered for no fertility indications.

ART

In principle IVF is not an indication for anovulation and that's exactly the case with PCOS. But we think about going for IVF when weight reduction, CC induction, low dose gonadotropins and even LOS fail. Single embryo transfer following controlled ovarian stimulation prevents the dreaded complications like OHSS and multiple pregnancies.

IVF is also indicated when other associated pathologies like tubal factor, male factor, severe endometriosis or peri-implantation diagnosis is indicated.

The best protocol till date is an antagonist protocol with freeze all and a freeze thaw single embryo transfer.

It has to be kept in mind that even after choosing the best and safest individualized protocol, your cycle can be cancelled (12.8% vs 4%) and duration of stimulation may be longer.

The probability of pregnancy is almost same as other non-PCOS patients and is around 35%.

IUI (Assisted Reproductive Technology)

Not a preferred choice
- Induction of ovulation in combination with IUI is indicated in women with PCOS and associated male factor infertility and may be proposed in women with

PCOS who fail to conceive despite successful induction of ovulation.

- Currently, double insemination does not appear to enhance the probability of pregnancy as compared with single IUI.

IVF and ICSI- Should be kept as the last option when ovulation induction is not achieved and risk for OHSS is too high. We stimulate, freeze all the embryos and then prepare the endometrium next cycle and thaw the embryos and transfer preferably one or two at a time.

Overall options look bleak from distance but if managed properly, PCOS woman have almost equal chance of getting pregnant and having a family of the size as their non-PCOS friends have.

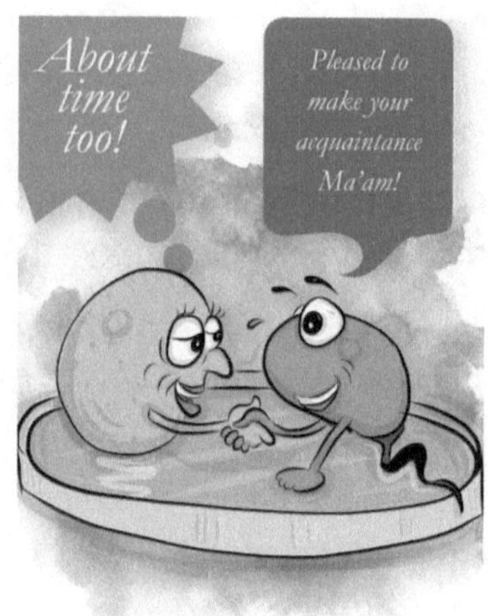

IVF treatment helps those who are unable to conceive naturally or with ovulation induction.

Chapter 21

Ultrasound in PCOS

Dr. Amitha Indersen, Dr. Pratik Tambe

"The more you praise and celebrate your life, the more there is in life to celebrate."
Oprah Winfrey

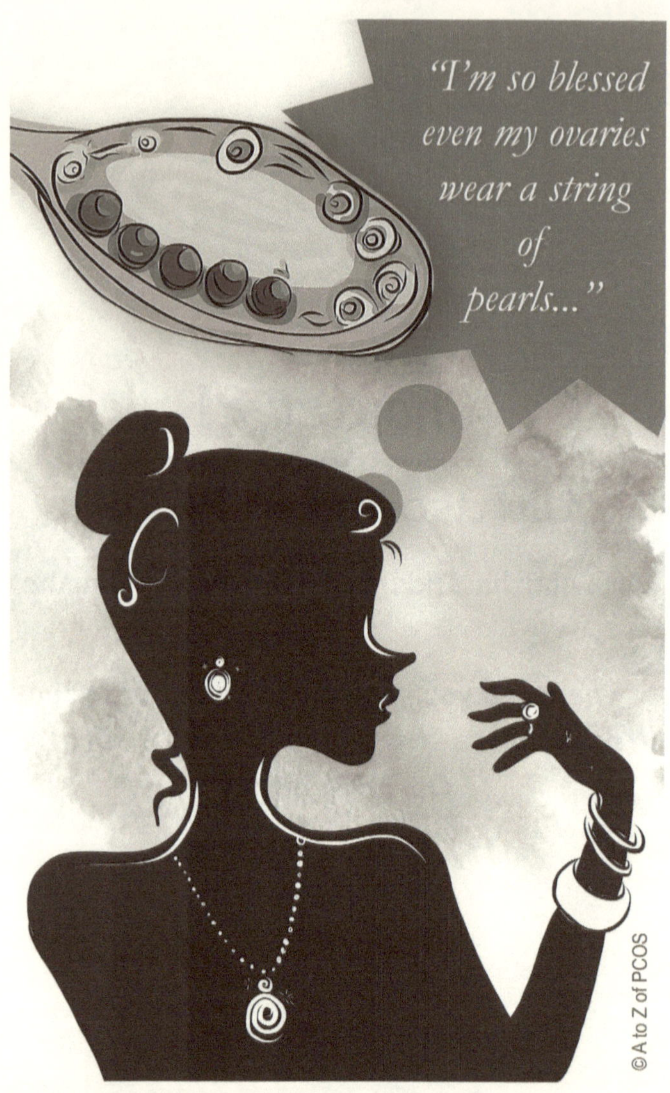

Having a positive attitude towards your problems can help you fight them better

It was a routine hectic Saturday and we were trying to keep the ultrasound clinic going at a steady pace and not prolong the patients' waiting period any longer than necessary. The next patient on our list was a Mrs Nidhi, a thirty two year old woman who had been married for 6 months and had a history of irregular menstrual cycles, right from when she was around nineteen years old. She had minimal hirsutism and her BMI was 30. So far she had not consulted a doctor regarding the irregular cycles and was not on any treatment. But now as she was planning to conceive she was going through the pre-conceptual check-up and wanted to have her periods regularized. Her blood tests were awaited. The scan was being done on Day 2 of her menstrual cycle which was ideal.

Mrs Nidhi had been asked to fill her bladder prior to the scan. This allowed us to screen the uterus and ovaries abdominally first. If the ovaries were large, high up in the pelvis or had large cysts it would be easier to visualize this abdominally. After that she was asked to empty her bladder completely and a vaginal scan was done. This is preferable in all women who have commenced sexual activity as it gives us better visualization of the pelvic organs with better precision and clarity. When the scan is done abdominally, the patient's body habitus, presence of gas in the bowel and poor penetration of sound waves make it technically difficult to image the ovaries.

On the ultrasound, the uterus looked normal in size with the musculature being normal. The endometrium or the uterine lining was much thickened but otherwise normal.

On imaging the ovaries both of them were enlarged, with multiple subcentimetre follicles. These follicles were arranged around the periphery of the ovary and formed what is called the necklace pattern. The tissue in the centre of the ovary called as the stroma appeared bright due to thickening of the stroma.

According to the widely used Rotterdam criteria for labeling the ovaries as polycystic, the following criteria have to be identified:

1. Enlarged ovaries with ovarian volume more than 10 cubic cm.

2. Multiple follicles present each measuring within 2–9mm and number more than 12 in each ovary.

3. The follicles were seen arranged in a Necklace Pattern in the periphery of the ovarian stroma.

4. The ovarian stroma or the ovarian tissue within appears thickened and echogenic (bright) due to thickening of the stroma.

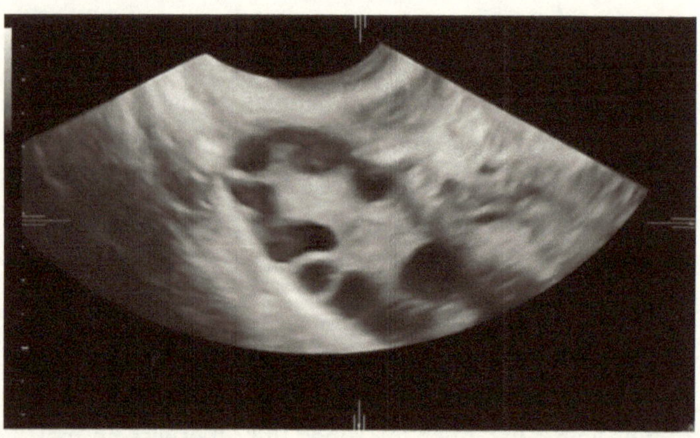

Ultrasound picture of Polycystic Ovary

Unless these criteria are satisfied we cannot label a person to be having polycystic ovaries. Unfortunately, in many places just the presence of a few follicles is reported as polycystic ovaries and is managed for the same. This is an over diagnosis.

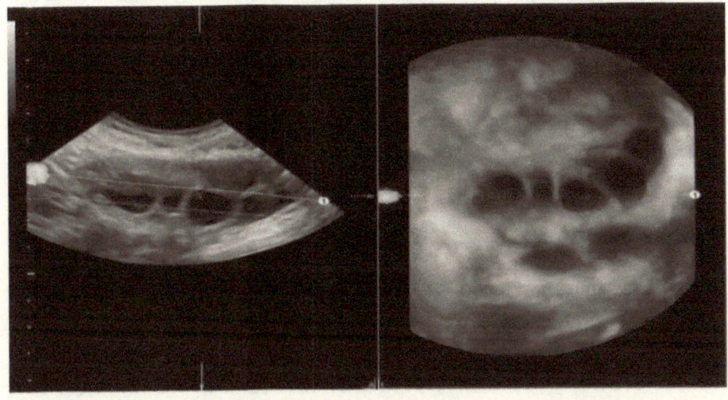

In women with polycystic ovaries and who are planning to conceive or have been trying to conceive it is important to look for the antral follicular count. Normally the ovary has hundreds of dormant egg cells and in every monthly cycle, a few are recruited and developed into follicles. In polycystic ovaries multiple egg cells are recruited in each cycle and in turn the baseline number of egg cells also decreases. By counting the antral follicles, we will be estimating the number of follicles that will be recruited for a particular cycle. If there are too many, the patient runs a risk of being hyperstimulated if medications are given to promote egg development and release. On the other hand, if the antral follicular count is low, it may be an indicator that the baseline pool is depleting or that the ovary may not respond very well to the ovulation induction drugs.

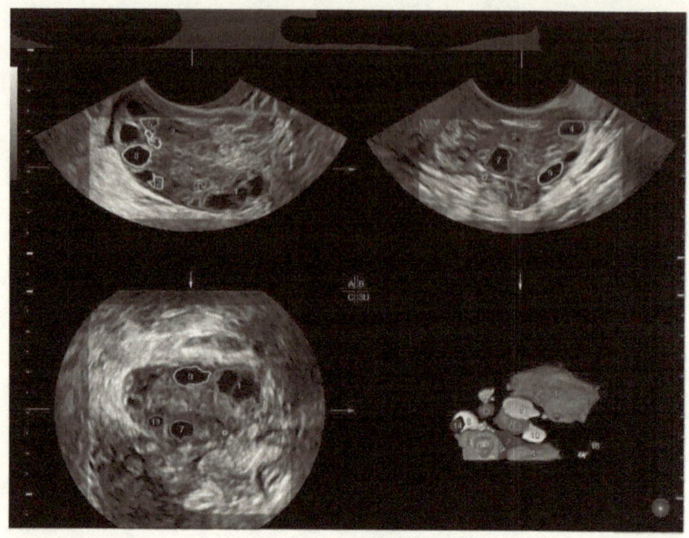

Antral Follicle Count

To conclude, Ultrasound is important to diagnose PCOS but the mere presence of few follicles is not PCOS and you may have PCOS even if the ultrasound is normal if you have the other features of menstrual disturbances and features of hyperandrogenism.

Chapter 22

Vit D Deficiency and PCOS

Rajalaxmi Walavalkar

"Let us dance in the sun, wearing wild flowers in our hair..."
Susan Polis Schultz

I think it's worth getting that tan, if it helps me fight my PCOS.
©A to Z of PCOS

Mrs Ruksar, a twenty four year old lady entered my office complaining of severe backache and which especially increased during her menstrual period. Those days were like hell for her. She was in good shape. She said that she went to the gym regularly and tried to keep herself fit, but her menses were scanty or sometimes they went haywire. And it was taking a toll on her work. She was absent from work for 3–4 days every month. She was quite worried about it. I realized she needed counseling first.

I spoke to her for almost 15 minutes and found out that she used to be in office throughout the day and during evenings she was a socialite; a party girl. So considering her issue, she was being asked to do routine investigations, hormonal profiles and ultrasonography. As expected, her hormonal profile showed deranged FSH and LH levels, ultrasonography showed polycystic pattern and Vitamin D3 less than 20pg/ml. So with this profile she was being labeled as PCOS and Vitamin D3 deficient.

So our discussion headed towards PCOS. It was important for me to make her understand what PCOS was. So I explained her that this was polycystic ovarian syndrome, which is composed of many diseases. It's because of her lifestyle, rather our modern lifestyle. This syndrome can be found in almost every 2nd or 3rd girl/women around us. In this syndrome, hormonal profiles get deranged, levels of vitamins like Vit. D3 gets lowered. Ultrasonography showed, typical black necklace pattern of ovary which meant that she had many small follicles in her ovary which were not grown or ruptured. Some patients experience unnecessary facial hair growth, voice changes, mood swings and importantly subfertility. PCOS patients are divided in two categories as thin PCOS and Obese PCOS.

She was prescribed OC pills for 6 months and Vitamin D3 in powder form as weekly dosages for 8 weeks and then to maintain stores once a month for a year. I asked her to take out 15 minutes daily to walk in sunlight, without thinking about getting tanned. And it was important to check on her diet, so a dietician's reference was taken. She was given her calcium, vit D3 rich, PCOS patient diet.

After two months, I got a call from Ruksar. She was on her holiday. While relaxing there she remembered me, as all her backache and dysmenorrhea had gone, like some magic. She was happy and enjoying herself. I asked her to continue in same vein.

Polycystic ovary syndrome (PCOS) is the most common endocrine disorder in women of reproductive age, presenting in up to 18% of this population. PCOS is characterized by the presence of polycystic ovaries, menstrual dysfunction, infertility and biochemical (elevated androgens) and clinical (hirsutism and/or acne) hyperandrogenism. PCOS is also associated with an increased incidence of cardiovascular disease (CVD) risk factors, including an increased prevalence of subclinical atherosclerosis, type 2 diabetes, dyslipidaemia and impaired glucose tolerance. Obesity and insulin resistance are closely linked to the development of PCOS and its clinical features.

It's becoming a major public health problem.

A number of studies have demonstrated associations between vitamin D levels and various PCOS symptoms, including insulin resistance, infertility and hirsutism. Vitamin D is thought to influence the development of PCOS through gene transcription, and hormonal modulation influences insulin metabolism and fertility regulation.

Several studies have reported low levels of vitamin D in women with PCOS, with an average of 25-hydroxy vitamin D (25OHD) levels between 11 and 31 ng/ml, with the majority having values <20 ng/ml.Vitamin D deficiency. It is also common in the general population in many parts of the world, with 10–60% of adults having values lower than 20 ng/ml. In general, vitamin D deficiency disrupts the function of all the systems of the body and increases the risk of chronic disease, including physical diseases such as cancer, cardiovascular, autoimmune and infectious diseases and psychological disorders such as depression and chronic pain.

Vitamin D3 is obtained from the diet or synthesized endogenously through sunlight-induced photochemical conversion of cholesterol to 7-dehydrocholesterol in the skin and subsequently hydroxylation in the liver and kidney.

A recent study in women with PCOS also found out that low vitamin D3 levels were significantly determined by the degree of adiposity (BMI and total fat mass) and were not directly affected by the development of insulin resistance. It is possible that the high prevalence of vitamin D deficiency in women with PCOS is related to obesity as vitamin D is fat soluble and in obesity, a higher proportion is sequestered in adipose tissue, lowering bioavailability. Alternatively obese subjects may spend less time outdoors exposed to sunlight that can lead to insufficient vitamin D biosynthesis in skin. It is also possible that dietary preferences and vitamin D metabolism may differ between obese and non-obese individuals.

Two small uncontrolled intervention studies have indicated that vitamin D therapy may have a beneficial effect on insulin resistance and insulin secretion in obese women with PCOS.

There is accumulating evidence that vitamin D plays an important role in reproductive function. Receptors have been found in the ovary, endometrium and placenta. Vitamin D deficiency is associated with calcium dysregulation, which contributes to the development of follicular arrest in women with PCOS and results in menstrual and fertility dysfunction.

Some researchers found relationship between vitamin D3 and reproductive function, with low levels of serum vitamin D3 being associated with ovulatory and menstrual irregularities. Higher vitamin D levels were associated with an increased likelihood for successful pregnancies, and there is evidence for a beneficial effect of vitamin D supplementation on menstrual dysfunction. Further evidence is needed to determine whether vitamin D supplementation is beneficial for pregnancy.

There is a relationship between vitamin D and hyperandrogenism. It has been suggested that the correlations between vitamin D status and hyperandrogenism may be due to the reduction in SHBG that results from obesity.

So overall it shows that vitamin D is associated with PCOS and it should be a part of PCOS treatment, irrespective of fertility issue.

Chapter 23

What risk do women have with PCOS?

Dr. Kumudini Chauhan

"Find a place inside where there is joy, and the joy will burn out the pain"
Joseph Campbell

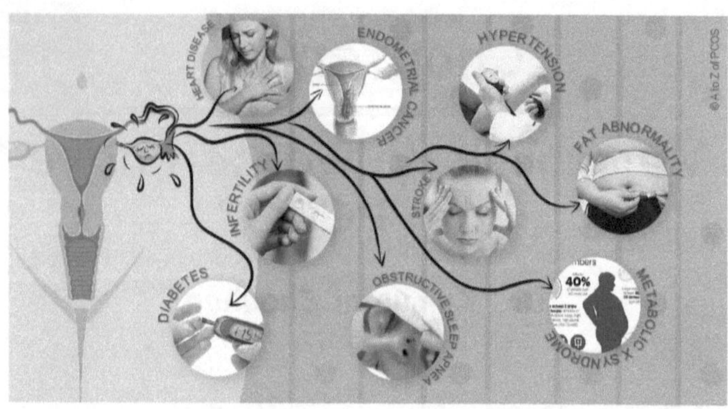

Women with PCOS are at greater risk of multiple problems but all can be averted and managed by proper attention, early detection and awareness.

What Risk Do Women Have With PCOS?

Does PCOS put women at risk for other health problems?

Women with PCOS have greater chances of developing serious health conditions, including life threatening diseases:

- More than 50% will have diabetes or prediabetes (impaired glucose tolerance) before the age of 40.

- The risk of heart attack is 4–7 times higher than in women of the same age without PCOS.

- There is a greater risk of having high blood pressure.

- Women with PCOS have high levels of LDL (bad) cholesterol and low levels of HDL (good) cholesterol.

- Can develop sleep apnea (when breathing stops for short periods of time during sleep).

- May develop anxiety and depression.

- At risk for endometrial cancer. Irregular menstrual periods and the lack of ovulation cause women to produce the estrogen, but not the progesterone. Without progesterone, the endometrium becomes thick, which can cause heavy or irregular bleeding. Over time, this can lead to endometrial hyperplasia, and cancer.

How does PCOS affect a woman while pregnant?

Women with PCOS appear to have higher rates of:

- Miscarriage

- Gestational diabetes

- Pregnancy-induced high blood pressure

- Premature delivery

Babies born to women with PCOS have a higher risk of spending time in a neonatal intensive care unit or of dying before, during, or shortly after birth. Metformin can be given to those who have insulin resistance and do not appear to cause any major birth defects or other problems during pregnancy. Metformin also lowers male hormone levels and limits weight gain in women who are obese when they get pregnant.

Does PCOS change at menopause?

Yes and no. PCOS affects many systems in the body. Many symptoms may persist even though ovarian function and hormone levels change as a woman nears menopause, such as, excessive hair growth continues, and male pattern baldness or thinning hair gets worse after menopause. Also, risks of complications from PCOS, such as heart attack, stroke, and diabetes, increase as a woman gets older.

Now you can nicely understand what is PCOS and what are the risk factors for PCOS. Previously PCOS was termed as PCOD which means Poly Cystic Ovarian Disease but now the word disease has been replaced with syndrome. As the name suggests this syndrome is associated with multiple health problems. If your gynecologist has diagnosed you with PCOS, then it is very important to understand the short-term and long-term health risks associated with this syndrome. *Not all women with PCOS will develop all of these conditions, but having PCOS does increase your risk for having these conditions.*

Why to know about them: *AWARENESS IS THE KEY*

If you are aware enough regarding these conditions, then you can prevent or delay before risks become diseases. Regular scheduled health check-ups are of prime importance for prevention and early diagnosis of these health problems so that we can treat them before they are full-blown. Check-up should be done by a gynecologist who has a good experience in treating PCOS women.

How long to continue check-ups: *PREVENTION IS BETTER THAN CURE*

It is important to continue regular monitoring even after menopause because long-term health problems associated with PCOS generally develop after 4th decade of life. Research is going on to develop screening guidelines in case of PCOS. Till then at least you should follow what your PCOS expert advises you.

Health risks

Fertility Problems: Infertility (inability to conceive) and subfertility (reduced fertility) are commonly associated with PCOS due to problem in egg formation. PCOS is the commonest cause of infertility secondary to problematic egg formation. Many times PCOS is diagnosed only when the woman consults the doctor for infertility.

Endometrial Cancer: Women with PCOS are at a high risk for developing uterine cancer. This happens due to infrequent periods during which uterine lining gets thicker (endometrial hyperplasia) and due to infrequent egg release and the unopposed action of estrogen hormone does harmful changes on the uterine lining which is supposed to be opposed by progesterone hormone as in case of normal menstrual cycle. This is the reason for which woman with PCOS needs to take progesterone pills to shed thickened uterine lining in case of amenorrhea.

Diabetes: You already have learned about how insulin resistance and diabetes is related with PCOS. So even you have normal sugar level today, you need regularly follow-up especially after 40 years of age.

Lipid Abnormality: If you are diagnosed as PCOS then start cutting fatty food from your diet because you are at high risk of developing dyslipidemia. Dyslipidemia is characterized by elevated levels of bad low density lipoproteins, cholesterol and decreased levels of good high density lipoproteins. This altered ratio of LDL and HDL lead to deposition of fat in blood vessels and increased risk of cardiovascular disorders.

Hypertension: In PCOS women, high blood pressure develops in the earlier decade than the normal population.

Heart attack: Evidences suggest increased risk of heart attack and other cardiovascular diseases in PCOS population. Tendency of obesity also adds to the risk as it does in non-PCOS obese population.

Stroke: Associated lipid abnormality and hypertension increase the risk of brain stroke.

Obstructive Sleep Apnea: This is characterized by pause in breathing during sleep, which can lead to waking episodes and restlessness. This is likely related to central obesity and insulin resistance. However some research showed that risk of sleep apnea is 30–40 folds higher in PCOS women compared with weight matched controls.

Genetic transmission: There is evidence that mothers and sisters of women with PCOS are more likely than the general population to have PCOS as well. Fathers and brothers of women with polycystic ovaries appear to be at increased risk for developing insulin resistance and type 2 diabetes. This indicates some level of genetic transmission. Hence family members of PCOS women should also go for check-up and screening procedure of related disease.

Conclusion

There should be national screening guidelines for health risks which are associated with PCOS because features of Asian PCOS population vary from PCOS of other part of world like we are at high risk of developing diabetes than others. As there are no guidelines we should follow the advice of a PCOS expert. Point of utmost importance is to know about your problem and tackle them before it becomes a disease.

Chapter 24

Metabolic X Syndrome and PCOS

Dr. Vimee Bindra

"The human body has been designed to resist an infinite number of changes and attacks brought about by its environment. The secret of good health lies in successful adjustment to changing stresses on the body."

Harry J. Johnson

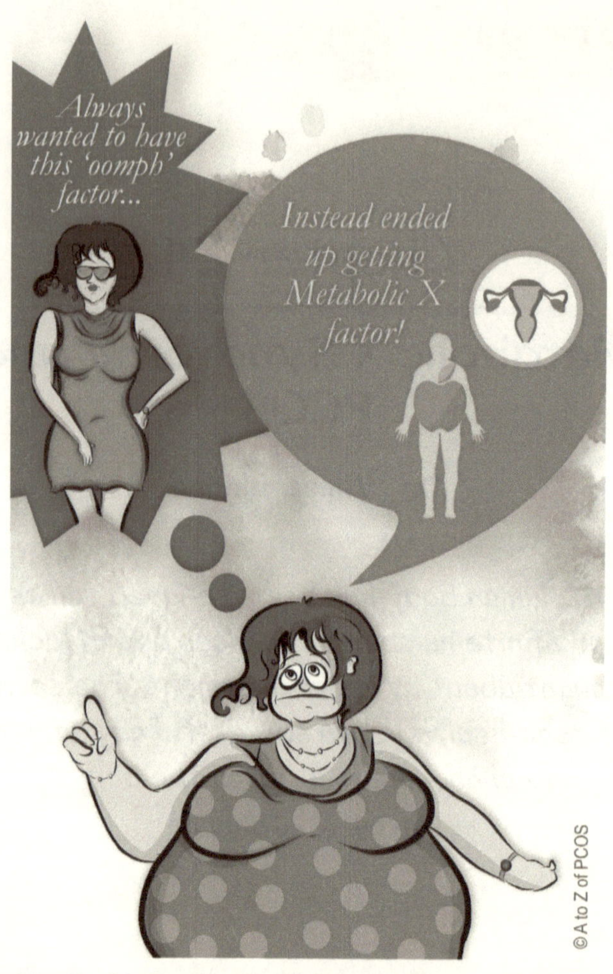

Oh My Gosh! Syndrome within Syndrome (Metabolic X Syndrome in Polycystic Ovarian Syndrome). Now what the hell is this?

Metabolic syndrome is the name for a group of risk factors that raises your risk for heart disease and other health problems, such as diabetes and stroke.

The five conditions mentioned below are the metabolic risk factors. You must have at least three of five for you to be diagnosed with metabolic syndrome.

1. A big waistline or abdominal obesity

2. High Triglyceride levels (Triglyceride is a type of fat in blood.)

3. A low HDL cholesterol (HDL is also referred to GOOD cholesterol which protects our heart as well.)

4. High blood pressure (or normal blood pressure but you are on medication to control blood pressure)

5. High blood sugar (or normal blood sugar and you are on diabetic medications)

Approximately one-third to one-half of all women and adolescent girls with polycystic ovary syndrome (PCOS) have the metabolic syndrome associated with increased risk for cardiovascular disease and type 2 diabetes.

Have you ever wondered what the common link between the two is? Is there a glue for them?

Yes the name of glue is **Insulin Resistance**. Insulin Resistance causes an imbalance of glucose and insulin levels, which impairs the vital process whereby glucose is converted into energy by passing through the cell wall via insulin.

The cell walls become desensitized to insulin by Insulin Resistance, with the result that much glucose is denied access to the cell and, instead it freely floats in the bloodstream, which takes it to the liver. Once there, the glucose is converted to fat and distributed around the body, where it can cause excess weight gain and lead to a variety of serious disorders, including PCOS, heart disease and certain forms of cancer.

Insulin Resistance also causes unhealthy levels of insulin in the body, which can lead to the onset of Pre- and type 2 diabetes, which, themselves, are increased risk factors for blindness, kidney disease and the need for amputation.

Because insulin resistance and visceral obesity are important features of polycystic ovary syndrome (PCOS), metabolic syndrome is much more common in women with PCOS than in the general female population of similar age. It has been reported that in the USA almost 50% of women with PCOS present the metabolic syndrome. Patients with mild PCOS phenotype (ovulatory PCOS) have a lower prevalence of metabolic syndrome but, in these patients too, metabolic syndrome is 2 times more frequent than in the normal population. These data suggest that PCOS is the most common cause of increased cardiovascular risk in young adult women. All obese and overweight women with PCOS should be screened for metabolic syndrome and, when the syndrome is not found, the screening should be repeated every 2 or 3 years. Treatment consists in lifestyle intervention. Medical therapies should be used only when lifestyle fails to normalize cardiovascular risk factors.

Chapter 25

Why Not Try Alternative Therapies for PCOS?

Dr. Vimee Bindra

"Meditate, Breathe consciously. Listen, pay attention, treasure every moment. Make the connection."
Oprah Winfrey

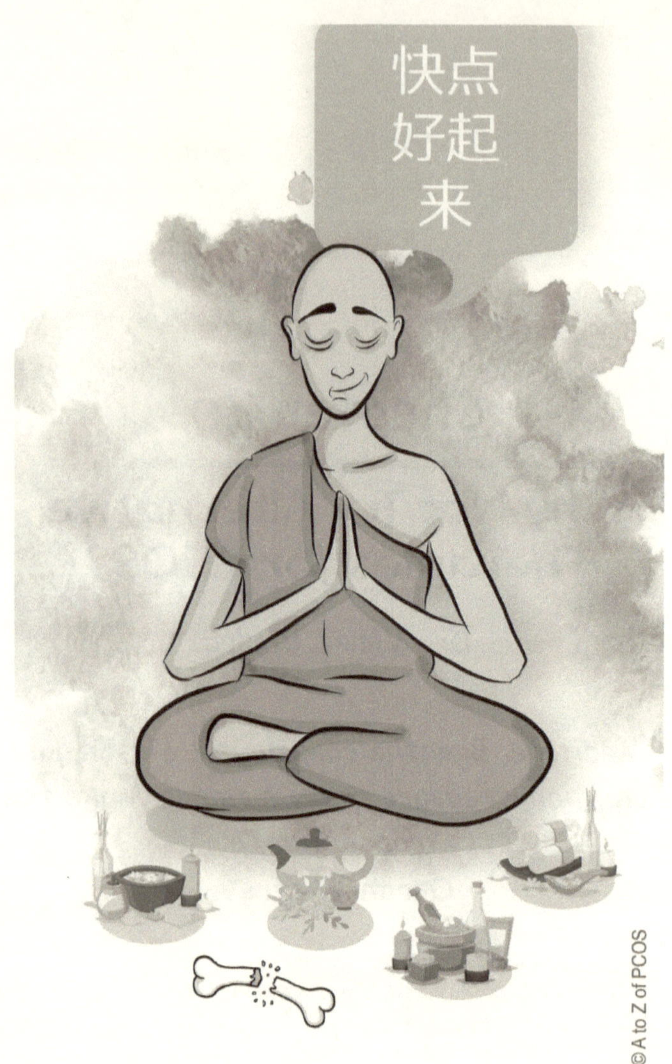

When women with PCOS do not get any relief with regular treatments, they do seek help of alternative medicine.

Mrs Rashmi was suffering from PCOS for the last five years with irregular cycles, weight gain and she was unable to conceive with various modalities of treatment with ovulation inducing agents and injectables. She was getting depressed and frustrated following different doctors' advice and taking several shots of injectables. One day, she met her friend after a long time and told her situation and she wanted some solution to this. Her friend knew somebody who treated PCOS for many patients with herbal treatment and acupuncture. Rashmi was convinced and thought of giving it a try. She discussed with her doctor and he said, "As such there is no evidence at present that it helps in healing PCOS but if you want, you can try, as in some studies it has shown some benefit."

Rashmi thought of trying it once and she took acupuncture therapy for three months and to everybody's surprise, she had regular cycles and within six months she got a positive pregnancy test.

Does that mean Absence of evidence is a sufficient evidence of non-existence?

Alternative therapy is emerging as one of the commonly practiced medicines for different health issues including PCOS.

Electroacupuncture (EA) study done in China also reported that EA enhances embryo quality in patients undergoing IVF probably by enhancing serum and follicular stem cell factor and another study showed EA improves spindle quality in oocyte hence enhances pregnancy rates in patients undergoing IVF-ET.

Some studies have also shown that combined therapy with clomiphene, Acupuncture and herbal medicine gives better pregnancy rates and less miscarriage rates.

Women with PCOS will have needles placed along the acupuncture meridians related to the reproductive system. This will help stimulate the organs, improve blood flow to the area, contribute to normalizing hormone levels, and promote the proper functioning of the reproductive system.

Thus far, only a limited number of RCTs have been reported. At present, there is insufficient evidence to support the use of acupuncture for treatment of ovulation disorders in women with PCOS

Recently published study has shown Durian (Durio zibenthinus Linn) a fruit of southeast Asia, is used as a natural supplement in healthy diets. Review studies have shown its effectiveness for metabolic syndrome but the effect on ovulation and fertility in PCOS is yet to be studied. The traditional use of this fruit as a fertility enhancing agent has to be studied by separating its components and ascertaining its fertility enhancing properties.

Use of Chinese herbal medicine, Cinnamon improves menstrual cyclicity in women with polycystic ovary syndrome. Results of a small randomized trial have shown improvements in menstrual cycles and can be considered as a treatment option.

Use of Amino acids, extracts and anti-oxidants has shown to decrease insulin resistance in PCOS. With this result demonstrated, it is necessary to modify the diet and to offer alimentary support to avoid the oxidative stress that impairs the insulin signaling with the subsequent insulin resistance.

Oral Carnitine administration has shown to reduce body weight and insulin resistance in patients with PCOS. In a randomized placebo controlled trial, oral administration of carnitine for 12 weeks resulted in reduction of weight, BMI, waist circumference, and also showed beneficial effects on glycemic control. However, it did not affect the lipid profile or testosterone levels.

Zinc supplementation for 50mg per day for 8 weeks had shown beneficial effects on alopecia, excessive hair growth but it did not improve overall hormonal profile.

Vitamin D deficiency and PCOS are interrelated. In a study where calcium and Vit D supplements were given to patients with PCOS, it has shown beneficial effects on inflammatory factor and biomarkers of oxidative stress.

D-chiro-Inositol has been shown in few studies to have modulatory role on LH and insulin secretion in obese PCOS. It helps restoring better insulin sensitivity and an improved hormonal pattern in obese hyperinsulinemic PCOS patients and in particular, in hyperinsulinemic PCOS patients who have diabetic relatives.

D-chiro- inositol has a cousin called as Myoinositol. Both are derivatives of inositol. Both of them have been shown to have beneficial effects in improving ovarian function and metabolism in patients with PCOS, although myo-inositol showed the most marked effect on the metabolic profile, whereas D-chiro-inositol reduced hyperandrogenism better.

Omega-3 fatty acids had some beneficial effects on serum adiponectin levels, insulin resistance and lipid profile in PCOS patients and may contribute to the improvement of metabolic complications in these patients.

Alternative medicine has been emerging as one of the commonly practiced medicines for different health problems. Alternative medicines include many modalities, such as kinesiology, herbalism, homeopathy, reflexology, acupressure, acupuncture, and massage therapy. Acupuncture is the most common modality.

PCOS is an enigma, its patho-physiology still not clearly understood. No treatment is a panacea, because treatments, so far, have been directed at the symptoms but not at the syndrome itself. Extensive efforts should be made to fully investigate the syndrome in order to make therapy more successful and to delay the serious long-term effects of the disease on patients' health.

Chapter 26

Zeal for life in PCOS

Dr. Seema Pandey

*"The key that unlocks energy is desire, it's
also the key to a long and interesting life,
if we expect to create any drive, any real
force within ourselves, we have
to get excited."*
Earl Nightingle

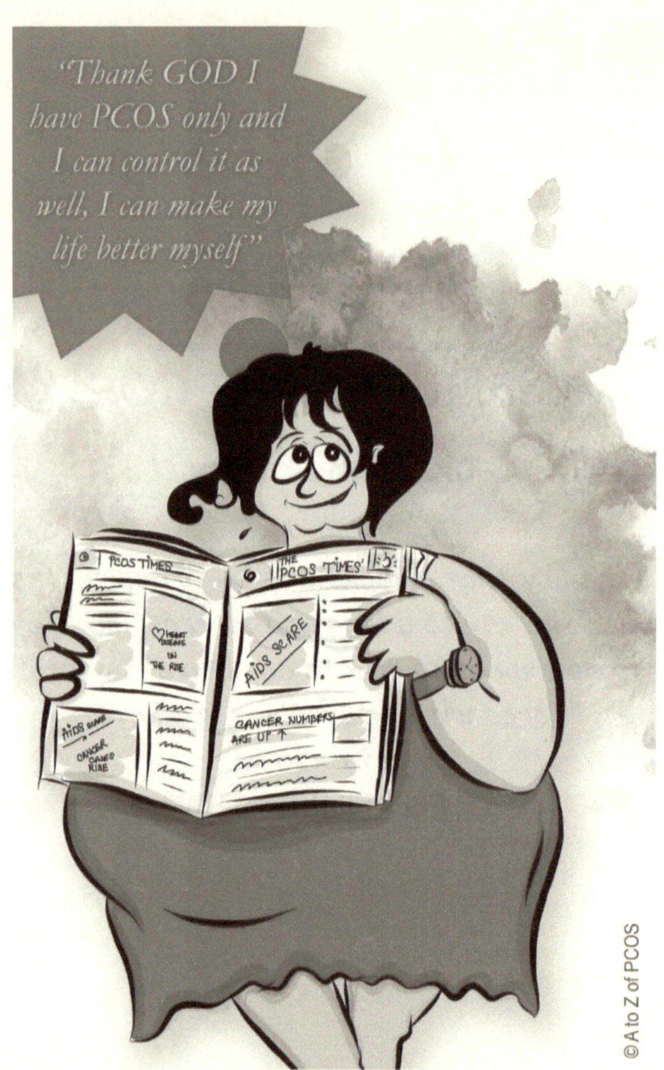

"Thank GOD I have PCOS only and I can control it as well, I can make my life better myself"
PCOS TIMES
THE 'PCOS TIMES'
HEART DISEASE ON THE RISE
AIDS SCARE
AIDS SCARE
CANCER CASES RISE
CANCER NUMBERS ARE UP
© A to Z of PCOS

As PCOS is a disorder which starts at a young age and lasts till menopause, it's obvious that a woman who has to face it throughout her life may get depressed or start feeling different. To prevent this feeling of desolation and stress, as it may further lead to cascade problems, one has to be enthusiastic and positive in dealing with PCOS. I remember two of my patients, one of them were obese with really deranged hormonal profile and a family who always used to press her for a child while the other one was of normal BMI range with mild symptoms and a very supportive husband. The reason I remember these two girls who were almost the same age was, whenever this healthy girl Saima would be in my clinic, her infectious laugh would create a positive atmosphere and she would chatter nonstop and will keep advising people to laugh and will always repeat, 'ma'am if I stop laughing will my disease get cured earlier?' And the day she understood her problem, she hugged me tight saying, "Thank God ma'am it's not like TB or Cancer, all I have to do is become cautious of what I eat and how I eat. Regarding my weight, you don't worry I will shed it off in a wink." Though her weight did not decrease much, but to my surprise she conceived in the third month of her treatment. I was pleasantly surprised as I could never imagine an obese PCOS like her getting pregnant so easily. On the other hand this pretty girl Pooja who I never saw smiling and whose doting husband would do anything to bring a smile on her lip, would ovulate regularly and despite all the other factors being normal, was not conceiving and getting more depressed. Then one day, when both of them were sitting in front of me, my brain started analyzing both of them subconsciously and it concluded that the winning shot for Saima was her zeal, enthusiasm and positivity for life which Pooja clearly lacked.

Maintaining this positivity and zeal is really difficult when you are facing one or the other problem ever since you remember but at the same time it's a key to success. Many women with hirsutism, acne and obesity feel less feminine or out of the league and for them it's important that they hear or see people who are facing similar problems and how are they coping. Whenever I get a few young girls on the same day of my appointment I try to introduce them to each other and encourage them to talk to each other as, in our country and especially in smaller places, you don't get proper and formal support groups. These girls, when they talk to each other, they realize that they are not alone in this and sometimes understand their problems better and the next time when they come to see me they are full of energy and enthusiasm. The key point in this is that you are the boss here and you can control your symptoms by changing the way you think, the way you eat and the way you lead your life.

These support groups, they are good and bad at the same time, while you read the positive stories you feel elated but some negative ones make you feel depressed. This support can come from the family as well, whenever I suggest some dietary and lifestyle modifications, I try to involve the husband or parents also, this involvement goes a long way and the girl will not feel secluded completely.

Few known support groups online are, PCO care foundation (www.pcosfoundation.org), PCOS awareness association (www.pcosaa.org), soul cysters (soulcysters.com) and PCOS challenge (www.pcoschallange.com).

Last but not the least if you really want to be happy nobody can stop you.

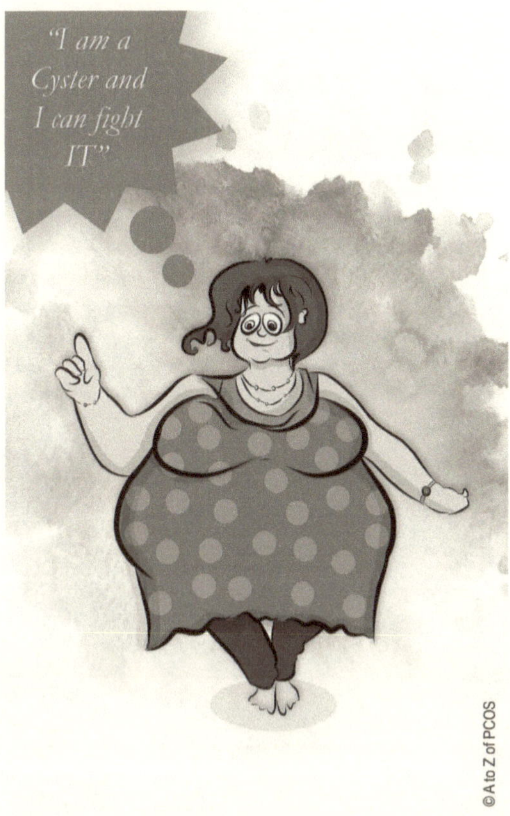

**Find the warrior within you and listen to what she says:
I am free, I am cosmic, I can change, I am my own brand
of beautiful, I am calm, I am grounded. I am a field of
wild flowers. I am ecstasy, I am capable. I am confident. I
can follow through. I am electric and empowered. I am a
winner. I am messy and perfect. I can make outstanding
decisions. I am not my parents or my society. I am an
alchemist, creator, and magic maker. I am love. I am the
sparkle in the darkest dark. I am me and it is enough.**

Thug Unicorn by Tanya Markul

About the Authors

Dr. Vimee Bindra

Dr. Vimee Bindra is a well-known gynecologist, fertility specialist and laparoscopic surgeon from Hyderabad, India. She has a special interest in research and management of PCOS. She lives in Hyderabad and works with Apollo Hospitals. She has won various academic awards at undergraduate and 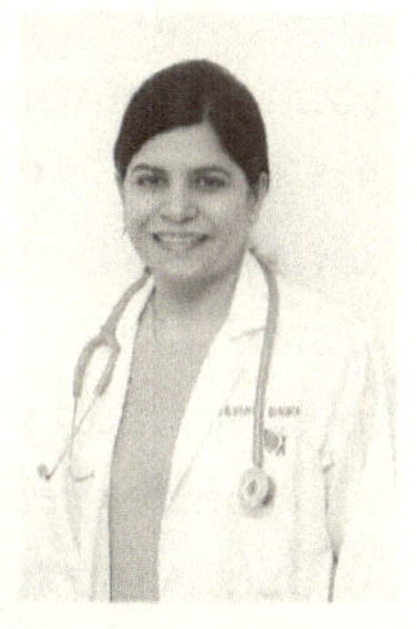 post-graduate levels. She has a keen interest in the field of Gynecological Endoscopy and Fertility-enhancing surgeries. She has vast surgical experience in different types of laparoscopic and hysteroscopy surgeries and PCOS-related infertility. Along with her medical education, she has done Masters in Hospital Administration (MHA) from ICFAI. She has presented various scientific papers in conferences at state and national levels and has also entered her name in Indian and International journals. She is an author of two well-known medical books in the field of Gynecology and Obstetrics by leading medical publishers of India. She regularly contributes chapters and articles for medical books and health magazines. She has a good command over five languages – English, Hindi, Bengali, Punjabi and Telugu. She is a surgeon par excellence and has done many difficult gynecological surgeries. Her aim of writing this book was to educate and empower women suffering from PCOS to lead a healthy and beautiful life.

Dr. Seema Pandey

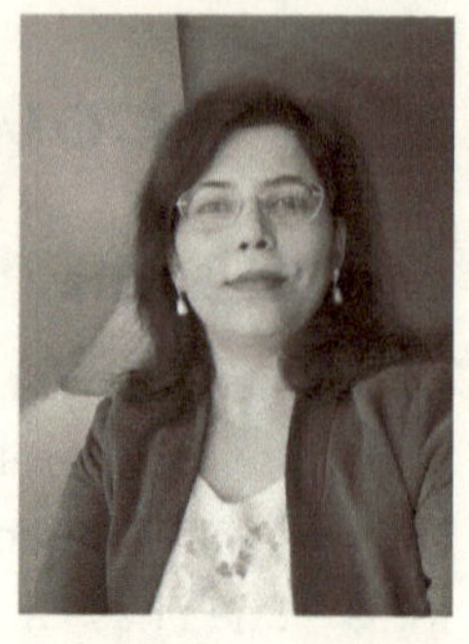

Dr. Seema Pandey is a well-known practicing reproductive medicine and infertility specialist for the last fifteen years. She has always been interested in medical research and social upliftment. And that passion for working at the grass root levels of society had brought her to Azamgarh District of Uttar Pradesh after completing her fellowships in reproductive medicine, laparohysteroscopy and ultrasonology. She runs her IVF and laparoscopy centre here. To pursue her academic interest, she keeps contributing her research work, articles and chapters in various national and international journals and reproductive medicine books. To keep herself updated and exchange knowledge, she keeps participating in various conferences nationally and internationally. PCOS and infertility are her passions and she not only treats it but through her NGO, she also works at schools among adolescent girls and pregnant mothers in villages and creates awareness about the disease and how, by changing their lifestyle, they can control it. Reading and writing are Dr. Seema's other hobbies.